**Pocket Guide to
Gastrointestinal Drugs**

Pocket Guide to Gastrointestinal Drugs

Edited by

M. Michael Wolfe, MD

Chair, Department of Medicine
MetroHealth Medical Center;
Charles H. Rammelkamp, Jr. Professor of Medicine
Case Western Reserve University School of Medicine
Cleveland, OH, USA

Robert C. Lowe, MD

GI Fellowship Director
Boston Medical Center;
Associate Professor of Medicine
Boston University School of Medicine
Boston, MA, USA

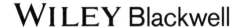

WILEY Blackwell

This edition first published 2014 © 2014 by John Wiley & Sons, Ltd.

Registered office:
John Wiley & Sons, Ltd, The Atrium, Southern Gate, Chichester, West Sussex, PO19 8SQ, UK

Editorial offices:
9600 Garsington Road, Oxford, OX4 2DQ, UK
The Atrium, Southern Gate, Chichester, West Sussex, PO19 8SQ, UK
111 River Street, Hoboken, NJ 07030-5774, USA

For details of our global editorial offices, for customer services and for information about how to apply for permission to reuse the copyright material in this book please see our website at www.wiley.com/wiley-blackwell

Library of Congress Cataloging-in-Publication Data

Pocket guide to gastrointestinai drugs / edited by M. Michael Wolfe, Robert C. Lowe.
  p. ; cm.
Includes bibliographical references and index.
  ISBN 978-1-118-48157-8 (paperback)
I. Wolfe, M. Michael, editor of compilation.   II. Lowe, Robert C., 1966- editor of compilation.
[DNLM: 1. Gastrointestinal Agents–therapeutic use–Handbooks.   2. Gastrointestinal Agents–pharmacology–Handbooks.   3. Gastrointestinal Diseases–drug therapy–Handbooks. QV 39]
  RM365
  615.7'3–dc23
                                                                                                2013041991

A catalogue record for this book is available from the British Library.

Wiley also publishes its books in a variety of electronic formats. Some content that appears in print may not be available in electronic books.

Cover image: iStock #10849434 © Mordolff
Cover design by Meaden Creative

Set in Palatino LT Std 9/12 pt by Aptara Inc., New Delhi, India

1   2013

Contents

List of contributors

Uri Avissar, MD
Boston Medical Center
Assistant Professor of Medicine
Boston University School of Medicine
Boston, MA, USA

Samra S. Blanchard, MD
Associate Professor
Division Head, Pediatric Gastroenterology and Nutrition
University of Maryland School of Medicine
Baltimore, MD, USA

Wanda P. Blanton, MD
Assistant Professor of Medicine
Section of Gastroenterology
Boston Medical Center
Boston University School of Medicine
Boston, MA, USA

Andrew K. Burroughs, MB. BCh Hons, FEB, FEBTM, Hon DSc (Med), FRCP, FMedSci
Consultant Physician and Hepatologist
The Royal Free Sheila Sherlock Liver Centre
Royal Free London NHS Foundation Trust;
Professor of Hepatology
Institute for Liver and Digestive Health
University College London
London, UK

Andrés Cárdenas, MD, MMSc, AGAF
Faculty Member and Senior Specialist
Institute of Digestive Diseases and Metabolism
University of Barcelona
Hospital Clinic
Barcelona, Spain

Raymond T. Chung, MD
Director of Hepatology, Medicine Service
Massachusetts General Hospital;
Associate Professor of Medicine
Harvard Medical School
Boston, MA, USA

Steven J. Czinn, MD
Professor and Chair, Department of Pediatrics
University of Maryland School of Medicine
Baltimore, MD, USA

James S. Dooley, BSc, MB, BS, MD, FRCP
Emeritus Reader in Medicine
Institute for Liver and Digestive Health
University College London;
Consultant Hepatologist
The Royal Free Sheila Sherlock Liver Centre
Royal Free London NHS Foundation Trust
London, UK

Douglas Drossman, MD
Adjunct Professor of Medicine and Psychiatry
University of North Carolina;
Co-director Emeritus
University of North Carolina Center for Functional GI and Motility
  Disorders
Drossman Center for the Education and Practice of Biopsychosocial Care
Chapel Hill, NC, USA

Francis A. Farraye, MD, MSc
Clinical Director, Section of Gastroenterology
Boston Medical Center;
Professor of Medicine
Boston University School of Medicine
Boston, MA, USA

Ronnie Fass, MD
Professor of Medicine Care, Western Reserve University;
Director, Division of Gastroenterology and Hepatology
Head, Esophageal and Swallowing Center
MetroHealth Medical Center
Cleveland, OH, USA

Gerald M. Fraser, MD, FRCP
Associate Professor of Medicine
Director, Inflammatory Bowel Disease Unit

Division of Gastroenterology
Rabin Medical Center
Beilinson Hospital
Petah Tikva;
Sackler Faculty of Medicine
Tel-Aviv University
Tel-Aviv, Israel

Albena Halpert, MD
Assistant Professor of Medicine
Section of Gastroenterology
Boston Medical Center
Boston University School of Medicine
Boston, MA, USA

Esther Jacobowitz Israel, MD
Assistant Professor, Pediatrics Harvard Medical School;
Director, Inpatient Quality and Safety
Associate Chief, Pediatric Gastroenterology and Nutrition
Mass General Hospital for Children
Boston, MA, USA

Savio John, MBBS
Assistant Professor of Medicine
SUNY Upstate
Syracuse, NY, USA

Hemangi Kale, MD
Assistant Professor of Medicine
Case Western Reserve University;
Fellowship Program Director
Division of Gastroenterology and Hepatology
MetroHealth Medical Center
Cleveland, OH, USA

Karen L. Krok, MD
Associate Professor of Medicine
Penn State Milton S. Hershey Medical Center
Hershey, PA, USA

Angel Lanas, MD, PhD
Chair, Digestive Diseases Service
University Hospital, IIS Aragón
University of Zaragoza, CIBERehd
Zaragoza, Spain

Lev Lichtenstein, MD
Senior Physician
Inflammatory Bowel Disease Unit
Division of Gastroenterology
Rabin Medical Center
Beilinson Hospital
Petah Tikva, Israel

Robert C. Lowe, MD
GI Fellowship Director
Boston Medical Center;
Associate Professor of Medicine
Boston University School of Medicine
Boston, MA, USA

Hannah L. Miller, MD
Assistant Professor of Medicine
Section of Gastroenterology
Boston Medical Center
Boston University School of Medicine
Boston, MA, USA

Christopher J. Moran, MD
Instructor in Pediatrics
Harvard Medical School;
Assistant in Pediatrics
Mass General Hospital for Children
Boston, MA, USA

David P. Nunes, MD
Director of Hepatology
Boston Medical Center;
Associate Professor of Medicine
Boston University School of Medicine
Boston, MA, USA

Melissa Osborn, MD
Associate Professor of Medicine
Division of Infectious Diseases
MetroHealth Medical Center
Case Western Reserve University
Cleveland, OH, USA

Dominic N. Reeds, MD
Assistant Professor of Medicine
Division of Geriatrics and Nutritional Science
Washington University School of Medicine
St. Louis, MO, USA

Joachim Richter, MD
Adjunct Professor of Tropical Medicine
University Hospital for Gastroenterology,
    Hepatology and Infectious Diseases
Heinrich-Heine-University
Düsseldorf, Germany

Carlos Sostres, PhD
Research Faculty
Digestive Disease Service
University Hospital, IIS Aragón
Zaragoza, Spain

Kentaro Sugano, MD
Chief Professor, Division of Gastroenterology
Department of Medicine
Jichi Medical University
Shimotsuke, Tochigi, Japan

Christina M. Surawicz, MD
Professor of Medicine
Department of Medicine
Division of Gastroenterology
Washington University School of Medicine
Seattle, WA, USA

Beth Taylor MS, RD, CNSC, FCCM
Nutrition Support Specialist
Barnes-Jewish Hospital
St. Louis, MO, USA

Gert Van Assche, MD, PhD
Professor of Medicine
University of Leuven
Leuven, Belgium;
Division of Gastroenterology
University of Toronto;
Division of Gastroenterology
Mount Sinai Hospital
Toronto, ON, Canada

M. Michael Wolfe, MD
Chair, Department of Medicine
MetroHealth Medical Center;
Charles H. Rammelkamp, Jr. Professor of Medicine
Case Western Reserve University School of Medicine
Cleveland, OH, USA

Preface

In the mid-1970s, Sir James Black developed the first H_2-receptor antagonist, cimetidine, a remarkable achievement that revolutionized the treatment of acid-peptic disorders and led to the awarding of his Nobel Prize in Medicine. One year after its approval by the US Food and Drug Administration in 1977, cimetidine became the most widely prescribed drug in the world. Three other H_2-receptor antagonists were subsequently marketed worldwide, and in the late 1980s, the first proton pump inhibitor omeprazole was approved for use and likewise became the most prescribed drug worldwide. Since that time, there has been a virtual explosion in the number of pharmaceutical agents available for the treatment of gastrointestinal diseases, from new biologic immunomodulators for inflammatory bowel disease to novel antiviral agents for the treatment of hepatitis B and C.

This handbook has been carefully formulated and written to provide the busy clinician with a concise, yet scholarly, review of the major classes of drugs used in the treatment of gastrointestinal and hepatobiliary disorders. Each chapter discusses the pharmacology and clinical effectiveness of classes of medications, including indications for use, dosing, and adverse events. The outstanding group of authors who have contributed their wisdom and experience represent academic centers from around the world, with contributions from Europe, Asia, and North America. The authors were selected primarily for their record of excellence as investigators, clinicians, and educators. All are engaged in clinical or basic investigation and are particularly proficient in the application of basic scientific information to the realm of patient management.

The target audience for this handbook includes gastroenterologists, gastrointestinal surgeons, and all physicians who care for patients afflicted with digestive disorders. The authors have used great care and discrimination in presenting their materials, and the subject matter has been composed in a concise, yet thorough, format. Accordingly, medical students, internal medicine, family medicine, and surgery residents, and gastroenterology fellows will view this guide as an invaluable adjunct to their educational needs, and it should be regarded as useful to the practices of emergency room and primary care physicians, hospitalists, intensivists, pharmacists, and other health care providers involved in the management of diseases of the gastrointestinal tract and hepatobiliary systems. While generic drug names are used throughout the text, each chapter also lists the international trade names for each drug to enable rapid identification of each agent.

We, the editors, dedicate this book to our colleagues and trainees, whose contributions to clinical care, research, and teaching have made our academic careers intellectually challenging and personally rewarding. We also thank Claire Brewer and Oliver Walter at Wiley, who approached the formidable task of publishing this handbook with the utmost care and who provided immeasurable assistance and advice throughout the course of formulating the content and producing the final product.

M. Michael Wolfe and Robert C. Lowe

UPPER GI TRACT

PART I

CHAPTER 1
Prokinetic agents and antiemetics

Hemangi Kale and Ronnie Fass
MetroHealth Medical Center, Cleveland, OH, USA

Prokinetics

Introduction

Prokinetic agents enhance coordinated gastrointestinal motility by increasing the frequency and/or the amplitude of contractions without disrupting normal physiological pattern and rhythm of motility.

Acetylcholine is the principle immediate mediator of muscle contractility in the GI tract. However, most clinically useful prokinetic agents act "upstream" of acetylcholine, at receptor sites on the motor neuron itself, or even more indirectly, on neurons that are one or two orders above. Acetylcholine itself is not pharmacologically utilized because it lacks selectivity. It acts on both nicotinic and muscarinic receptors and is rapidly degraded by acetylcholinesterase. Dopamine is present in significant amounts in the GI tract and has an inhibitory effect on motility. It reduces both lower esophageal sphincter basal pressure and intragastric pressure. These effects are mediated by D_2 receptors through suppression of acetylcholine release from myenteric motor neurons. Thus, dopamine receptor antagonists are effective prokinetic agents because of antagonizing the inhibitory effect of dopamine on myenteric motor neurons. Additionally, they act centrally on the chemoreceptor trigger zone (CTZ), thereby relieving nausea and vomiting. Presently, very few prokinetics are available in the market, primarily due to the failure of many of these compounds to demonstrate significant symptom improvement when compared with placebo in pivotal indication trials. In addition, these agents have an unacceptable safety profile. The exact reasons for the former are unknown but are believed to be related to disassociation between severity and/or frequency of symptoms and the severity or even the presence or absence of a motility abnormality.

Pocket Guide to Gastrointestinal Drugs, Edited by M. Michael Wolfe and Robert C. Lowe. © 2014
John Wiley & Sons, Ltd. Published 2014 by John Wiley & Sons, Ltd.

Metaclopramide (Reglan)

Metaclopramide is indicated for the prophylaxis of chemotherapy-associated nausea and vomiting (second line agent); diabetic gastroparesis; gastroesophageal reflux disease (GERD); prior to endoscopic or radiologic exam, to place a feeding tube beyond the pylorus; and postoperative nausea and vomiting. Metaclopramide is also commonly used, but not FDA approved in, nondiabetic gastroparesis, hyperemesis gravidarum, and dyspepsia.

Mechanism of action

The drug works through several mechanisms. It is a dopamine receptor antagonist, a 5-HT$_3$ antagonist, and a 5-HT$_4$ agonist. It also blocks serotonin receptors in the chemoreceptor trigger zone of the central nervous system (CNS). Metaclopramide enhances the response to acetylcholine in the upper GI tract, resulting in coordinated contractions and thus accelerated gastric emptying, as well as increasing lower esophageal sphincter tone.

Pharmacology

Metaclopramide is absorbed rapidly after oral ingestion, metabolized by the liver and is excreted principally in the urine with a t ½ of 4–6 hours. The onset of action after oral administration is 30–60 minutes; after IV administration, 1–3 minutes; and after IM administration, 10–15 minutes. Dosing of metaclopramide for each different indication is listed in Table 1.1. The bioavailability of different medications may be affected due to accelerated gastric emptying. Drugs with narrow therapeutic indices need to be monitored closely when administered concomitantly with metoclopramide. The concomitant administration of CNS depressants, such as anxiolytics, hypnotics or sedatives, as well as alcohol, with metoclopramide can possibly increase sedation. The concomitant administration of metoclopramide with drugs that can cause extrapyramidal reactions is contraindicated. Patients with hepatic impairment do not need dosage adjustment. In addition, patients with mild renal impairment (CrCl ≥40 ml/minute) do not require a dosage adjustment. However, patients with CrCl <40 ml/minute require a dose reduction of 50%.

Adverse effects

Major side effects due to central dopamine antagonism include extrapyramidal reactions, such as acute dystonic attack, pseudo-parkinsonism, akathisia, tardive dyskinesia, and rarely neuroleptic malignant syndrome. Parkinson-like symptoms occur several weeks after the initiation of therapy and usually subside 2–3 months after the discontinuation of

Table 1.1 Dosing and route of administration of metaclopramide (Reglan)

Indications	Adult dosage	Child dosage
Diabetic gastroparesis	Oral: 10 mg 30 minutes before each meal and bedtime for 2–8 weeks Parenteral: IV/IM: 10 mg if oral route is not available	
IV infusion for chemotherapy-induced emesis	1–2 mg/kg administered over 15 minutes, beginning 30 minutes prior to chemotherapy and repeated as needed every 2–3 hrs	1–2 mg/kg administered over 15 minutes, beginning 30 minutes prior to chemotherapy and repeated as needed every 2–3 hrs
Post-operative nausea/vomiting and nausea vomiting prophylaxis	10 mg IM or IV near end of the surgical procedure, repeat every 4–6 hrs as needed	0.1–0.2 mg/kg IV, repeat every 6–8 hrs as needed
Gastroesophageal reflux disease (GERD)	10–15 mg orally up to 4 times/day. Therapy – recommended no more than 12 weeks	Child/infant: 0.1 mg/kg orally 3–4 times/day Neonates: 0.15 mg/kg orally every 6 hrs
Prior to endoscopic or radiologic procedures	10 mg IV	<6 years: 0.1 mg/kg IV single dose; 6–14 years: 2.5.5 mg IV

therapy. Tardive dyskinesia can occur after weeks to years of therapy initiation and may be irreversible. It appears to be more common in elderly patients. Strategies such as titrating to lowest effective dose and drug holidays may decrease these side effects. Patients should be warned to inform their physician if any involuntary movements develop. Rarely, cardiac arrhythmias, hypersensitivity reactions, hyper-prolactinimia, impotence and neuroleptic malignant syndrome have all been reported.

Motilin agonists

Motilin, a peptide hormone found in the GI M cells and some enterochromaffin cells, is a powerful contractile agent of the upper gastrointestinal (GI) tract. Erythromycin and other macrolide antibiotics like azithromycin and clarithromycin mimic the molecular structure of motilin and thus are potent promotility agents. Rapid development of tolerance and side effects, as well as concerns about using antibiotics long term, limits the use of these drugs as prokinetics. Intravenous erythromycin may be used to "restart or kickstart" the stomach during acute episodes of gastroparesis. It has also been used to clear the stomach prior to endoscopy of patients with an upper gastrointestinal bleed.

Pharmacology
The standard dose of erythromycin for gastric stimulation is 3 mg/kg IV or 200–250 mg orally every 8 hours and for azithromycin 250 mg daily. For small intestinal motility, a lower dose of 40 mg IV is more commonly used. However, the drugs are contraindicated in concomitant use with astemizole, dihydroergotamine, ergotamine, pimozide, terfenadine and in patients with known hypersensitivity to motilides. In elderly patients with renal/hepatic impairment, there is an increased risk of hearing loss, hepatotoxicity and QT prolongation. Lastly, erythromycin has been designated as Pregnancy Category B.

Adverse effects
Gastrointestinal toxicity (nausea, anorexia, diarrhea, abnormal liver enzymes and jaundice), bacterial resistance, pseudomembranous colitis and sudden cardiac death due to prolonged QT interval syndrome have all been well documented. Azithromycin has similar effects on GI motility as the other macrolides but was originally thought to lack drug interaction that can lead to prolonged QT interval. However, the FDA recently issued a warning that azithromycin can lead to fatal arrhythmia in certain patients. The extent of the risk is unknown. The macrolides require adjustment in patients with hepatic impairment because of the possibility of accumulation, whereas in patients with renal impairment, no need for dose adjustment is necessary.

Bethanechol
Bethanechol is a prokinetic agent that improves GI motility by acting as a cholinergic agonist, releasing acetylcholine from nerve endings. The drug is less commonly used today as a prokinetic due to its high rate of cholinergic-related adverse events and poor patient tolerability. While not specifically indicated for GI-related disorders, the drug has been used in GERD, primarily in patients who are refractory to proton pump inhibitor (PPI) treatment. The dosing is 25 mg orally four times a day. Bethanechol is contraindicated in patients with asthma and bradycardia.

Its adverse effects are primarily related to its cholinergic effects and consequently also include syncope, dizziness, diarrhea, and urgent desire to urinate. Bethanechol is designated as Pregnancy Category C.

Domperidone

The drug is not FDA approved but is available in many countries outside the US, including Mexico and Canada. It is a peripheral dopamine D_2 receptor antagonist. It does not readily cross the blood brain barrier (BBB) and is hence less likely to cause extrapyramidal side effects. It can affect CNS areas that lack this barrier and those areas involved in temperature control, prolactine release and emesis. The drug is used for gastroparesis and GERD. The drug is dosed 10 to 20 mg three times a day.

Antiemetic agents

Introduction

Nausea (Latin *nausea*, from Greek vauoia, nausie, "motion sickness," "feeling sick," queasy" or "wamble") is a sensation of unease and discomfort in the upper abdomen, which often leads to vomiting. Vomiting, an act of forceful expulsion of stomach contents, is a complex process, consisting of coordination between central and peripheral mechanisms. Vomiting is coordinated by a central emesis center in the lateral reticular formation of the mid brainstem that is adjacent to both the chemoreceptor trigger zone (CTZ) in the area postrema (AP) at the base of the forth ventricle and the solitary tract nucleus (STN) of the vagus nerve. The absence of a BBB allows the CTZ to monitor blood and cerebrospinal fluid constantly for toxic substances and to relay information to the emesis center. It also receives input from the vagus nerve via the STN, splanchnic afferents via the spinal cord, the cerebral cortex and the vestibular apparatus. CTZ has high concentration of 5-HT_3, dopamine and opioids receptors, while the STN is rich in enkephalin, histamine, acetylcholine and 5-HT_3 receptors.

Antiemetics are classified according to the predominant receptor on which they are proposed to act. However, the mechanisms of action may overlap among the different antiemetics. Data comparing antiemetics in specific disorders is very limited; hence drug selection in a particular situation is empiric, based on preferred route of administration, safety and personal experience.

Five neurotransmitter receptor sites have been identified that play an important role in the vomiting reflex: muscarinic (M_1), dopamine (D_2), histamine (H_1), serotonin (5-HT_3), and Substance P/Neurokinin Receptor 1. Consequently, antiemetics were primarily developed as

Table 1.2 The different antiemetic classes

Antiemetic class	Medications	Common therapeutic utilization
5-HT$_3$ antagonist	Ondansetron (Zofran) Granisetron (Kytril) Dolasetron (Anzemet) Palonosetron (Aloxi)	Chemotherapy-induced nausea and vomiting prophylaxis Radiation-induced nausea and vomiting prophylaxis Postoperative nausea and vomiting prophylaxis
D$_2$ antagonist	Metoclopramide (Reglan) Prochlorperazine (Compazine) Trimethobenzamide (Tigan) Droperidol (Inapsine)	Chemotherapy-induced nausea and vomiting Motion sickness Postoperative nausea and vomiting
H$_1$ receptor antagonist	Cyclizine (Bonine for children, Marezine) Promethazine (Phenergan) Hydroxyzine (Atarax, Vistaril) Meclizine (Antivert, Bonine, Dramamine, Zentrip, VertiCalm)	Motion sickness Postoperative nausea and vomiting prophylaxis
M$_1$ antagonist	Hyoscine (Scopolamine)	Motion sickness
NK$_1$ antagonist	Aprepitant (Emend) Fosaprepitant (Emend Inj)	Chemotherapy-induced nausea and vomiting
Cannabinoids	Dronabino (Marinol) Nabilone (Cesamet)	Chemotherapy-induced nausea and vomiting

inhibitors of these receptors (Tables 1.2, 1.3 and 1.4). This chapter will not cover the serotonin-related products, which are discussed elsewhere in this book.

Dopamine receptor antagonists

Three classes of dopamine receptor antagonists are currently available. They include phenothiazines: prochlorperazine (Compazine), chlorpromazine (Thorazine); butyrophenones: droperidol (Inaspine), haloperidol (Haldol); and benzamides: metoclopramide (Reglan), Domperidone (Motilium) and trimethobenzamide hydrochloride (Tigan).

Table 1.3 Dosing and indications of antiemetic medications

Indication	Antiemetic class	Medications	Adult dose
Motion sickness	H_1 antagonists	Cyclizine	50 mg q4–6 hr. oral/IM Max 200 mg/24 hr 30 min. before travel
		Hydroxyzine	25–100 mg IM/PO q4–6 hr. Max 600 mg/day 30 min. before travel
		Meclizine	50 mg orally q24 hrs. Start 1 hour before travel
		Promethazine	25 mg orally BID 30 min. before travel
	M_1 antagonists (anticholinergics)	Scopolamine	1 transdermal patch behind ear 4 hours before travel. Replace every 3 days if needed.
Post-operative N/V	H_1 antagonists	Promethazine	12.5–25 mg orally/IM/IV q4–6 hrs Max. 50 mg/dose orally/IM; 25 mg/dose IV
		Cyclizine	50 mg IM/IV q4–6 hrs
	D_2 antagonists	Metoclopramide	10 mg IM or IV near end of surgical procedure Repeat q4–6 hrs as necessary
		Tigan	Adult: 300 mg orally q6–8 hrs 200 mg IM q6–8 hrs
		Compazine	Adult: 5–10 mg orally q6–8 hrs 5-10 mg IM or 2.5–10 mg IV q3–4 hrs 25 mg suppository rectally q12 hrs
		Droperidol	Adult: 0.625–1.25 mg IM/IV q3–4 hrs as needed Max 2.5 mg IM/IV May repeat 1.25 mg based on response, cautiously
	M_1 antagonists (anticholinergics)	Scopolamine	1 transdermal patch behind ear the evening before surgery and 24 hrs after

Table 1.4 Pregnancy class and use in children of antimetic medications

Antiemetic class	Medications	Pregnancy class	Use in children
D_2 antagonist	Metoclopramide (Reglan)	B	Yes
	Prochlorperazine (Compazine)	C	Yes (>2 years)
	Trimethobenzamide (Tigan)	C	No
	Droperidol (Inapsine)	C	Yes (>2 years)
H_1 receptor antagonist	Cyclizine (Bonine for children, Marezine)	B	Yes (>6 years)
	Promethazine (Phenergan)	C	Yes (>2 years)
	Hydroxyzine (Atarax, Vistaril)	C	Yes
	Meclizine (Antivert, Bonine, Dramamine, Zentrip, VertiCalm)	B	Yes (>12 years)
M_1 antagonist	Hyoscine (Scopolamine)	C	Yes
NK_1 antagonist	Aprepitant (Emend)	B	No
	Fosaprepitant (Emend Inj)	B	No
Cannabinoids	Dronabinol (Marinol)	C	No
	Nabilone (Cesamet)	C	No

Phenothiazines

The phenothiazines are the most commonly used antiemetics. These drugs are moderately effective for nausea caused by various GI and non-GI disorders and in mild to moderate, but not highly emetogenic, chemotherapy. Prochlorperazine (Compazine) predominantly blocks D_2 dopamine receptors in the area postrema, but also possesses muscarinic (M_1) and histamine (H_1) antagonist effects. Prochlorperazine is indicated for severe nausea and vomiting. Although not indicated, it is also used in chemotherapy–induced nausea and vomiting. The drug is contraindicated in children under 2 years of age, comatose states, and in patients with hypersensitivity to phenothiazines. The drug should be cautiously used in elderly patients with dementia-related psychosis, adolescents and children with signs suggestive of Reye's syndrome and in those with bone marrow suppression. The adverse effects include hypotension, hypertension, and prolonged QT interval.

Chlorpromazine (Thorazine) is used less often than prochlorperazine. It is a dimethylamine derivative of phenothiazine, whose exact mechanism of action is unknown. It has weak anticholinergic, antihistaminic and antiserotonin activities. The drug is indicated for nausea, vomiting and intractable hiccups. The dosing for nausea and vomiting in the adult is 10–25 mg orally every 4–6 hours and 25 mg IV/IM every 3–4 hours. In the pediatric population, the dose is 0.25 mg/lb orally and 0.125 mg/lb IM. Chlorpromazine is contraindicated in a comatose state, concomitant use of large doses of CNS depressants and in those with hypersensitivity to the drug. Administration in elderly patients with dementia-related psychosis or those with bone marrow suppression should be cautiously done. Adverse effects include akathesia, dizziness, tardive dyskinesia, and constipation. In patients with hepatic impairment, a lower dose should be considered. In contrast, in patients with renal impairment, there is no need for dose adjustment. The drug has been designated Pregnancy Category C.

Butyrophenones

The butyrophenones are used for procedural sedation as preanaesthetic agents and for post-operative nausea and vomiting. They are tranquilizers that potentiate action of opioids and have antiemetic effect when used alone.

The exact mechanism of action of droperidol (Inapsine) is unknown. Its antiemetic effect may be due to binding of GABA receptors in the CTZ. It antagonizes the action of dopamine by binding to D_2 receptors centrally. The drug is indicated for nausea and vomiting associated with surgical or diagnostic procedures and for prophylaxis of nausea/vomiting. The drug is not indicated, but is commonly used, for nausea and vomiting due to other reasons and for chemotherapy-induced vomiting. Droperidol is contraindicated in patients with hypersensitivity to the drug or those with prolonged QT interval. In those patients with other arrythmogenic medications, elderly patients, and in patients with renal or hepatic impairment, the drug should be used with caution. Adverse effects include prolonged QT interval, torsades de pointes, ventricular tachycardia, cardiac arrest, hypertension, and somnolence. In patients with hepatic impairment, lower doses may be required. Similarly, in patients with renal impairment, lower doses are required.

Benzamides

The benzamides include metoclopramide and domperidone, which are discussed earlier in this chapter.

Trimethobenzamide hydrochloride (Tigan) is a dopamine receptor antagonist that is indicated for nausea due to gastroenteritis and for postoperative nausea and vomiting. The drug is contraindicated in patients with previous hypersensitivity to the drug and in patients in the pediatric age group. Elderly patients may have an increased risk of extrapyramidal and CNS side effects. Adverse effects include hypotension, xerostomia, diarrhea, anticholinergic adverse reactions, and somnolence. A decrease in the total daily dose or frequency of administration should be considered in patients with diminished renal function, defined as a CrCl # 70 ml/minute. In those with hepatic impairment, there is no need for dose adjustment. In pregnant women, fetal risk cannot be ruled out.

Histamine 1 receptor antagonists

The antihistaminics are histamine 1 (H_1) receptor antagonists that are primarily useful for motion sickness and post-operative emesis. Their precise mechanism of action is not known, but may be due to a direct effect on the labyrinthine apparatus, as well as central action on CTZ.

Cyclizine (Marezine) is indicated in adults for nausea and vomiting due to motion sickness and should be taken 30 minutes prior to travel time. It is also indicated in the pediatric population for postoperative vomiting. The dose for those aged 6–12 years is 25 mg every 6–8 hours, not to exceed 75 mg/24 hours. For those older than 12 years, the dose is 50 mg every 4–6 hours, not to exceed 200 mg/24 hours. In patients with postoperative nausea who are between the ages of 6–10 years, the dose is 3 mg/kg/day in three divided doses IM or orally. The drug is contraindicated in patients with known hypersensitivity to the drug. In subjects with asthma, COPD, glaucoma, congestive heart failure (CHF), obstructive uropathy and epilepsy, caution should be taken when using the drug. Adverse effects include drowsiness, dizziness, dry mucous membranes, pancytopenia, arrhythmias, and heat stroke.

Hydroxyzine (Atarax, Vistaril) is indicated for motion sickness. In patients with renal impairment (CrCl <50), the dose should be decreased by 50%, while in those with hepatic impairment, the frequency of administration should be decreased. Another member of the antihistaminics family is promethazine (Phenergan). The drug is indicated for nausea/vomiting and for motion sickness. Dose adjustments have not been defined in patients with renal or hepatic impairment.

Meclizine (Antivert, Bonine, Dramamine, Zentrip), another H_1 antagonist, is used for non-GI related indications, but also for motion sickness.

Anticholinergic agents

Scopolamine is a belladonna alkaloid that possesses anticholinergic properties. It functions as an M_1-muscarinic antagonist by blocking cholinergic transmission from the vestibular nuclei. The drug is indicated for motion sickness and postoperative nausea and vomiting (1.5 mg transdermal patch). Scopolamine is contraindicated in COPD, liver impairment and in patients with tachyarrythmia. Adverse effects include xerostomia, blurred vision, and somnolence.

Neurokinin receptor antagonists

Aprepitant (Emend) and fosaprepitant (Emend Injection) are selective high affinity antagonists of human substance P/neurokinin 1 (NK_1). In animal models, they appear to work at the cerebral cortex and dorsal raphae. By inhibiting the substance P/neurokinin 1 receptor, they prevent acute and delayed vomiting. They are indicated for chemotherapy-associated nausea and vomiting due to highly and moderately emetogenic chemotherapy, nausea and vomiting prophylaxis and post-operative nausea and vomiting prophylaxis.

Aprepitant (Emend) is dosed for chemotherapy-induced nausea and vomiting prophylaxis at 125 mg orally 1 hour prior to chemotherapy on day 1 followed by 80 mg orally daily in the morning on days 2 and 3 (used in combination with corticosteroids/5-HT_3 antagonist as per treatment protocol). In postoperative nausea-vomiting prophylaxis, the drug is dosed at 40 mg orally once, 3 hours prior to anesthesia.

Fosaprepitant (Emend Injection) is dosed for chemotherapy-induced nausea and vomiting as a single-dose regimen, a single dose of 150 mg IV started 30 minutes prior to chemotherapy on day 1 or as a three-day regimen. An alternate regimen includes a single dose of fosaprepitant 115 mg IV, followed by aprepitant 80 mg orally for 2 days, which is started 30 minutes prior to chemotherapy. The drug is contraindicated in patients with hypersensitivity to the medication and those with severe liver impairment. Adverse effects may include neutropenia, bradycardia, and Stevens Johnson syndrome. In hepatic impairment, there is no dose adjustment for Child-Pugh A and B. However, it is not yet defined for C. There is no need for dose adjustment in renal impairment.

Cannabinoids

The exact mechanism of action of cannabinoids is not known, although they bind to cannabinoid receptors in the neural tissues. Dronabinol is indicated in chemotherapy-induced nausea and vomiting prophylaxis. The drug is dosed in adults at 5 mg/m^2 orally 1–3 hours before chemotherapy and 5 mg/m^2 orally every 2–4 hours after chemotherapy for total of 4–6 doses/day. The dose may be increased by 2.5 mg/m^2 to a maximum of 15 mg/m^2/dose. Nabilone7 is dosed in the adult at 1–2 mg orally 2–3 times a day, 1–3 hours prior to chemotherapy. The drug may be given the night before chemotherapy (1–2 mg). The maximum is 6 mg a day. Both drugs are not recommended to patients below age 18. They are contraindicated in those with hypersensitivity to dronabinol, cannabinoids and sesame oil. They should be used cautiously in patients with a history of alcohol abuse, seizure disorder and psychiatric illness. Adverse effects include tachyarrythmia, abdominal pain, amnesia and ataxia. No need for dose adjustments in patients with either hepatic or renal impairment.

Recommended reading

Glare PA, Dunwoodie D, Clark K, Ward A, Yates P, Ryan S, Hardy JR (2008) Treatment of nausea and vomiting in terminally ill cancer patients. *Drugs* **68**(18): 2575–90.

Hasler WL (2008) Management of gastroparesis. *Expert Rev Gastroenterol Hepatol* June; **2**(3): 411–23.

Hejazi RA, McCallum RW, Sarosiek I (2012) Prokinetics in diabetic gastroparesis. *Curr Gastroenterol Rep* Aug.; **14**(4): 297–305.
    A comprehensive review on the topic diabetic gastroparesis that also includes our present knowledge about prokinetics, antiemetics and future drug development.

Karamanolis G, Tack J (2006) Promotility medications – now and in the future. *Dig Dis* **24**(3–4): 297–307.
    An excellent review on the currently available prokinetics, as well as those that presently are undergoing clinical evaluation.

Olden KW, Chepyala P (2008) Functional nausea and vomiting. *Nat Clin Pract Gastroenterol Hepatol* Apr.; **5**(4): 202–8.

Reddymasu SC, Soykan I, McCallum RW (2007) Domperidone: review of pharmacology and clinical applications in gastroenterology. *Am J Gastroenterol* **102**(9): 2036–45.
    A nice review with a specific focus on domperidone, which includes pharmacology, clinical application and safety profile of the drug.

Sawhney MS, Prakash C, Lustman PJ, Clouse RE (2007) Tricyclic antidepressants for chronic vomiting in diabetic patients. *Dig Dis Sci* Feb.; **52**(2): 418–24.

Stapleton J, Wo JM (2009) Current treatment of nausea and vomiting associated with gastroparesis: antiemetics, prokinetics, tricyclics. *Gastrointest Endosc Clin N Am* Jan.; **19**(1): 57–72.
    Another comprehensive review of antiemetics and prokinetics in the treatment of gastroparesis. It also discusses the role of tricyclics in the treatment of nausea and vomiting.

Steele A, Carlson KK (2007) Nausea and vomiting: applying research to bedside practice. *AACN Adv Crit Care* **18**(1): 61–73.

CHAPTER 2
Proton pump inhibitors

Wanda P. Blanton[1] and M. Michael Wolfe[2]
[1]Boston University School of Medicine, Boston, MA, USA
[2]Case Western Reserve University School of Medicine, Cleveland, OH, USA

Introduction

Proton pump inhibitors (PPIs) are used clinically in the treatment of acid related disorders, including gastroduodenal (peptic) ulcers, gastroesophageal reflux disease (GERD), nonsteroidal anti-inflammatory (NSAID) induced gastroduodenal ulcers, stress-related ulcer syndrome in critically ill patients, Zollinger-Ellison syndrome (ZES), and as a component of *Helicobacter pylori* (*H. pylori*) eradication. Prior to the introduction of PPIs, histamine H_2-receptor antagonists (H2RAs) were the mainstay of therapy for these disorders. The introduction of PPIs in the 1980s expanded the therapeutic options and has allowed clinicians to optimize the medical treatment of these acid related disorders.

Mechanism of action, pharmacodynamics, kinetics

Parietal cells, which comprise ~85% of the cell population in the stomach, secrete 0.16 M hydrochloric acid (HCl) upon stimulation by acetylcholine, histamine, and gastrin (Figure 2.1). Upon meal stimulation, the parietal cell undergoes intracellular structural changes to increase the surface area of the cell to enable the active transport of H^+ ions against a 3 000 000:1 ionic gradient in exchange for K^+ (Figure 2.2). With the discovery that the final step in parietal cell acid secretion required an apical surface H^+/K^+ adenosine triphosphatase (ATPase) enzyme (Figure 2.1), PPIs were developed as specific inhibitors of this ATPase.

The PPIs function as prodrugs that share a common structural motif, a substituted pyridylmethylsulfinyl benzimidazole, but vary in terms of their substitutions, which yield slightly different pKa values. The prodrug is a weak protonatable pyridine that traverses the parietal cell membrane. As the prodrug accumulates in the highly acidic secretory canaliculus, it undergoes an acid catalyzed conversion to a reactive

Pocket Guide to Gastrointestinal Drugs, Edited by M. Michael Wolfe and Robert C. Lowe. © 2014 John Wiley & Sons, Ltd. Published 2014 by John Wiley & Sons, Ltd.

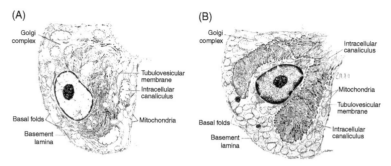

Figure 2.1 **(A)** Electron photomicrograph of parietal cell in the resting (unstimulated) state demonstrating abundant cytoplasmic tubovesicular membranes to which proton pumps – hydrogen potassium ATPase (H^+/K^+ ATPase) are inserted. **(B)** Stimulated parietal cell demonstrating translocation of the tubovesicular membranes (containing proton pumps) to the intracellular secretory canalicular membranes, facilitating pump exposure to the highly acidic canalicular lumen.

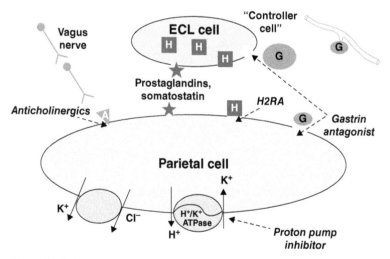

Figure 2.2 Schematic representation of the factors influencing gastric acid secretion by the parietal cell. A number of physiologic mechanisms affect acid secretion: neurocrine (acetylcholine and other neurotransmitters from vagal efferent neurons), paracrine (somatostatin from D-cells and histamine from gastric enterochromaffinlike cells), and endocrine (circulating gastrin) factors. Dashed arrows indicate potential sites of pharmacologic inhibition of acid secretion, either via receptor antagonism or via inhibition of H^+/K^+ ATPase. A, acetylcholine and other neurotransmitters; EGL, enterochromaffinlike; G, gastrin; H, histamine; PG, prostaglandin; S, somatostatin.

Source: Adapted from MM Wolfe and G Sachs (2000). Reproduced with permission of Elsevier.

species, the thiophillic sulfenamide. This active moiety then covalently binds to a specific cysteine residue (Cys 813) on the H^+/K^+ ATPase (via disulfide bond formation) and inactivates it, thus suppressing basal and stimulated gastric acid secretion. The rate of conversion to the active form varies among the PPIs, as activation occurs when the regional pH decreases below the pKa of the specific PPI. Thus, some PPIs may have a slightly faster onset of action, with rabeprazole having the most rapid onset (pKa 5.0), followed by omeprazole, lansoprazole, esomeprazole (pKa 4.0), and finally pantoprazole (pKa 3.9). These pharmacokinetic differences have not proven to be clinically significant.

The PPIs are the most potent inhibitors of gastric acid secretion available when administered correctly, based on their pharmacodynamics. Because acid secretion must be stimulated for maximum efficacy, PPIs should be taken before the first meal of the day. PPIs are most effective when administered after a prolonged fast, when the greatest number of H^+/K^+ ATPase molecules is present in parietal cells, which is in the morning for most patients. In addition, administration of PPIs should be followed by food ingestion, when the gastric parietal cells are stimulated to secrete acid in response to a meal. Moreover, these drugs should *not* be used in conjunction with H2RAs, prostaglandins, somatostatin analogs, or other antisecretory agents. Animal studies have demonstrated that the concomitant administration of PPIs and other antisecretory agents markedly reduces the acid inhibitory effects of PPIs. In most individuals, once-daily dosing is sufficient to produce the desired level of acid inhibition. A second dose, if required, should be administered before the evening meal. Importantly, meals should include protein or another stimulant of gastric acid secretion (e.g., coffee). In addition, based on the pharmacokinetics of PPIs, the most effective response occurs with consistent (i.e., daily) dosing, rather than sporadic (i.e., as needed) dosing.

The oral bioavailability of PPIs ranges from 45% (omeprazole) to 85% (lansoprazole). Although PPIs have a circulating $T_{1/2}$ of only 1–1.5 hours, the biological $T_{1/2}$ of the inhibited complex is ~24 hours, due to its mechanism of action. Because all the PPIs require accumulation and acid activation, their onset of inhibition is delayed, and after the initial dose, acid secretion continues, but at a reduced level. Subsequently, H^+/K^+ ATPase enzymes that are recruited to the secretory canaliculus in the parietal cell are then inhibited by additional doses of PPI, further reducing acid secretion. Steady state acid inhibitory properties occur by ~5 days and inhibit maximal acid output by 66%.

PPIs are principally metabolized by CYP2C19, a member of the hepatic cytochrome P450 family of enzymes, with the exception of lansoprazole, which is mainly metabolized by CYP3A4. It is possible that PPIs may affect the metabolism of other drugs that are metabolized by this family of enzymes, including warfarin, diazepam, phenytoin, digoxin, carbamazepine, and theophylline. Asian populations and the elderly commonly harbor polymorphisms in the *CYP2C19* gene, which affects PPI metabolism and has been shown to increase the drugs' acid inhibitory properties. PPIs are mainly excreted in urine, with the exception of lansoprazole, which is mainly excreted in feces.

Clinical use and dosing

PPIs are widely used and generally considered safe and effective. Six different compounds of proton pump inhibitors currently exist on the market. The specific brand names vary (Table 2.1), depending upon the country of sale, and include omeprazole, lansoprazole, rabeprazole, pantoprazole, esomeprazole, and dexlansoprazole. The first PPI approved for use in the United States was omeprazole, while pantoprazole was the first PPI approved for intravenous use in the USA. With the exception of omeprazole (pregnancy Class C), all PPIs have been categorized as Class B agents.

PPIs are used to treat a number of acid-related disorders, including acute gastroduodenal (peptic) ulcer, treatment and prevention of NSAID-associated ulcers, gastroesophageal reflux disease (GERD), medical management of Zollinger-Ellison syndrome prior to definitive surgical treatment, treatment and prevention of GI hemorrhage, stress ulcer bleeding in critically ill patients, and as a component in the treatment of *H. pylori* eradication. They are also commonly used to treat nonulcer dyspepsia.

Table 2.1 Links to proton pump inhibitor trade names	
	Dexilant, formerly Kapidex (renamed in the USA to avoid confusion with other medications)
Dexlansoprazole	http://www.takeda.com/news/2010/20100305_3748.html
Esomeprazole	http://bddrugs.com/product5.php?idn=5&prev=2&prev1=&prev2=
Lansoprazole	http://en.wikipedia.org/wiki/Lansoprazole#Brand_names
Omeprazole	http://www.egeneralmedical.com/rxlist00000053.html
Pantoprazole	http://bddrugs.com/product5.php?idn=7&prev=&prev1=&prev2=
Rabeprazole	http://en.wikipedia.org/wiki/Rabeprazole#Formulations_and_brand_names

Peptic ulcer disease (Table 2.2)

PPIs are the cornerstone of therapy for peptic ulcer disease (PUD) and demonstrate superior efficacy and rate of healing compared to H2RAs in a number of studies. In general, the duration of therapy for acute duodenal ulcers is 4 weeks, and 8 weeks for gastric ulcers. Although the pathogenesis of PUD is often multifactorial and a function of mucosal defense factors and aggressive factors (i.e., *H. pylori* infection, NSAID use, hypersecretory states), acid secretion plays a central role in ulcer formation, and thus remains the rational target for therapy. While PPIs heal gastroduodenal ulcers more rapidly than H2RAs, no significant differences in ulcer healing have been demonstrated among the various PPIs. A meta-analysis comparing the healing of duodenal ulcers (DU) demonstrated that omeprazole 20 mg every morning for four weeks was superior to both ranitidine 300 mg and cimetidine 800 mg, both administered at bedtime. Similarly, another meta-analysis found that lansoprazole 30 mg every morning healed significantly more ulcers than ranitidine 300 mg and famotidine 40 mg, both administered at bedtime. The pooled healing rates were 60 and 85% for lansoprazole at two and four weeks, respectively, while the corresponding figures for the H_2-antagonists were 40 and 75%. Both rabeprazole and pantoprazole have demonstrated superior and accelerated DU healing compared to H2RAs. PPIs also appear to heal gastric ulcers (GU) more rapidly and at a greater rate than H2RAs. For example, a study found that pantoprazole healed 32 and 15% more gastric ulcers at four weeks and eight weeks, respectively, compared to

Table 2.2 Recommended proton pump inhibitor doses in active and maintenance therapy of gastroduodenal ulcers* and primary and secondary prevention of NSAID**-induced ulcers

Proton pump inhibitor	Dose (adult) oral – all administered once daily before breakfast***
Dexlansoprazole	30–60 mg
Esomeprazole	20–40 mg
Lansoprazole	15–30 mg
Omeprazole	20–40 mg
Pantoprazole	20–40 mg
Rabeprazole	20 mg

*Recommended duration of treatment: active duodenal ulcers – treat for 4 weeks, and gastric ulcers – treat for 8 weeks.
**NSAID, nonsteroidal anti-inflammatory drug.
***Meals should contain protein to enhance parietal cell stimulation.

ranitidine. While clearly more effective, as will be discussed, the margin of benefit conferred by PPIs over H2RAs in the healing of ulcers is far smaller than the advantage offered by these agents in the treatment of GERD. Moreover, like H2RAs, the optimal duration of therapy with PPIs should be four and eight weeks of therapy for acute DU and GU, respectively.

NSAID-associated ulcers

In addition to the discontinuation of NSAID use whenever feasible, the optimal treatment of acute NSAID-induced ulcers includes PPIs. Two large, multicenter studies comparing PPI to misoprostol and PPI to H2RA showed that PPIs were as effective or more effective in healing ulcers and erosions and in improving symptoms associated with NSAID-induced ulcer treatment. In one study, comparing omeprazole and ranitidine in patients with gastroduodenal ulcers who continued their NSAID, ulcer healing rates at eight weeks were 79, 80, and 63% in those receiving 40 mg of omeprazole, 20 mg omeprazole, and ranitidine 150 mg twice daily, respectively. Another study compared the efficacy of lansoprazole and ranitidine in the healing of gastric ulcers in patients continuing NSAID therapy. After eight weeks, ulcers were healed in 57% of the individuals receiving ranitidine 150 mg twice daily, while healing rates were 73 and 75% in those treated with lansoprazole 15 mg and 30 mg (each once daily), respectively. These observations indicate that PPIs possess the capacity to heal gastroduodenal ulcers at an accelerated rate whether or not NSAIDs are continued.

Owing to the number and serious nature of NSAID-related GI complications, recent efforts have been directed at the prevention of mucosal injury induced by NSAIDs. Because dyspeptic symptoms are not a reliable warning sign for the development of serious NSAID-related mucosal injury, it is important to identify patients who are more likely to suffer adverse consequences with NSAID therapy. Risk factors for the development of GI mucosal injury associated with NSAID use include advanced age, prior history of ulcer, high dose of NSAIDs or multiple NSAID use, concomitant use of steroids and NSAIDs, concomitant use of anticoagulants and NSAIDs, and co-morbid conditions, such as cardiovascular disease, diabetes mellitus, or impaired renal or hepatic function. PPIs have also proven effective in both primary and secondary prevention of NSAID-related ulcers in many studies. Two double-blind, placebo-controlled, randomized multicenter studies (VENUS and PLUTO trials) examined the impact of using esomeprazole for ulcer prevention in at-risk ulcer-free patients taking NSAIDs. The pooled results of the study demonstrated significant reduction in ulcer rates compared to placebo – 16.5% on placebo versus 0.9% on esomeprazole (20 mg) and 4.1% on higher dose esomeprazole (40 mg). For secondary prevention, one study examined the prevention of recurrent gastroduodenal ulcer in arthritic individuals in whom ulcers had healed and NSAID therapy was continued. For this study, 432 patients were randomly assigned to treatment with either 20 mg of omeprazole once daily or 150 mg of ranitidine twice daily. At six months, 16.3 and 4.2% of those given ranitidine developed GU and DU, respectively, while only 5.2% developed a GU and 0.5% a DU in the omeprazole group. Another study compared the effects of omeprazole and misoprostol in preventing ulcer recurrence in arthritic individuals continuing NSAID therapy. It should be noted that misoprostol, a prostaglandin analog, was the first drug approved for this indication; it is used infrequently now because of its less optimal safety profile. In this double-blind, placebo-controlled trial, 732 patients in whom ulcers had healed were randomized to receive either placebo, 20 mg of omeprazole once daily, or 200 μg of misoprostol two times per day as maintenance therapy. After six months, DU was detected in 12 and 10% of those treated with placebo and misoprostol, respectively, while only 3% of those treated with omeprazole developed a DU. GU relapse occurred in 32, 10, and 13% of the individuals receiving placebo, misoprostol, and omeprazole, respectively. Numerous other studies have shown similar benefit with other PPIs, and no significant differences in ulcer healing have been demonstrated among the various formulations. Besides primary and secondary prevention of NSAID-associated ulcers, PPIs have also been shown to prevent and treat upper gastrointestinal dyspeptic and reflux symptoms in patients taking low dose aspirin (OBERON trial). These studies suggest that PPIs are superior to H2RAs in maintaining patients in remission during continued NSAID use, as well as in improving dyspeptic symptoms associated with their use.

Gastroesophageal reflux disease (Table 2.3)

Numerous studies have proven the efficacy of PPIs in controlling GERD symptoms and healing esophagitis. Pooled data from three studies including 653 patients treated with lansoprazole 30 mg daily in patients with Grade II or worse esophagitis showed 80–90% healing at 4 weeks and 92% healing at 8 weeks. Comparative trials of PPIs and H2RAs show a clear advantage with the former agents. One trial comparing lansoprazole 30 mg daily and ranitidine 300 mg twice daily in patients with moderate to severe erosive GERD showed 91% healing in 8 weeks with lansoprazole compared with 66% healing for ranitidine. PPIs are also effective in patients with GERD unresponsive to high-dose H2RA therapy. In patients refractory to cimetidine 800 mg four times daily or ranitidine 300 mg three times daily, therapy with omeprazole 40 mg in the morning healed esophagitis in 91% of patients studied. In

Table 2.3 Treatment of erosive or nonerosive gastroduodenal reflux disease

Proton pump inhibitor	Dose (adult) oral – all administered daily before breakfast; second dose if necessary should be given before evening meal
Dexlansoprazole	30 mg daily or 30 mg twice daily
Esomeprazole	20 or 40 mg daily
Lansoprazole	30 mg daily or 30 mg twice daily
Omeprazole	20–40 mg daily or 20 mg twice daily
Pantoprazole	40 mg daily or 40 mg twice daily
Rabeprazole	20 mg daily or 20 mg twice daily

general, standard doses of PPIs (omeprazole/esomeprazole 20–40 mg, lansoprazole/dexlansoprazole 30 mg, rabeprazole 20 mg, or pantoprazole 40 mg, all administered before breakfast) will relieve symptoms and heal esophagitis in approximately 85–90% of cases. A large meta-analysis of 43 randomized controlled trials comparing PPIs to H2RAs or placebo demonstrated aggregate healing rates of 84% for PPIs vs. 52% for H2RAs.

The available PPI formulations have demonstrated similar efficacy in head-to-head trials in the treatment of GERD. A meta-analysis of randomized controlled trials using PPIs to treat erosive esophagitis found no significant difference among omeprazole, lansoprazole, pantoprazole, and rabeprazole in control of heartburn symptoms and in rates of mucosal healing. A large randomized controlled trial (n=2425) compared esomeprazole to omeprazole in patients with erosive esophagitis. The former was associated with significantly greater rates of healing and control of symptoms than omeprazole (93.7% vs. 84.2%). This result is to be expected, given that esomeprazole contains only the active enantiomer found in omeprazole. In comparison with other PPIs, however, esomeprazole does not demonstrate clear superiority. A large study (n=5241) compared esomeprazole 40 mg po QD to lansoprazole 30 mg po QD in the treatment of erosive esophagitis. Healing rates with esomeprazole were 92.6% compared with 88.8% in the lansoprazole group. Although this difference was statistically significant, the absolute rates were very similar, underscoring the comparable clinical effectiveness of most PPI formulations.

Because GERD is a chronic disorder, maintenance therapy is an important issue in the management of patients with the diseases. Most patients with GERD, and especially those with Grade III and IV esophagitis, will relapse once therapy is discontinued. In addition, maintenance of remission usually requires the same type and dose of medication that initially healed the esophagitis. All studies have demonstrated significantly better remission rates with PPI therapy than with H2RAs or prokinetic regimens, and PPIs thus constitute the preferred maintenance therapy in most patients with GERD.

Zollinger-Ellison syndrome (ZES)

ZES consists of the clinical triad of peptic ulcerations, gastric acid hypersecretion and gastrin-secreting neuroendocrine tumors most commonly located in the duodenal wall and the pancreas. While the tumors grow slowly, patients most commonly nevertheless succumb to these malignancies. Prior to the discovery of PPIs and H2RAs, total gastrectomy was often the procedure of choice for refractory peptic ulcers. However, total gastrectomy for gastric acid hypersecretion in the present PPI era is now rarely performed. Patients with ZES should be treated initially with a PPI, using twice the dose normally employed to treat gastroduodenal ulcers associated with *H. pylori* infection or NSAID use (e.g., omeprazole or rabeprazole 40 mg, lansoprazole 60 mg, or pantoprazole 80 mg, all administered before breakfast).

The relief of epigastric pain does not reliably predict the absence of mucosal injury, and the only parameter proven to reliably predict gastroduodenal mucosal injury is the level of acid inhibition. After a steady state has been achieved, basal acid output (BAO) should ideally be measured one hour before the next dose of the PPI is to be administered. The goal of therapy is not achlorhydria, but rather a BAO of 1–10 mmol/h. If complete inhibition of acid secretion occurs, the PPI dose should be decreased by 50% and the patient reassessed. However, if the BAO exceeds 10 mmol/h, the PPI dose should be increased incrementally, and for doses greater than 60 mg of omeprazole (or an equivalent dose for the other PPIs), the PPI should be administered twice daily in equally divided doses before breakfast and dinner. Patients should be evaluated periodically (every 6–12 months) with dose adjustments made based upon basal acid output. In contrast to H2RAs, which are now rarely employed for the treatment of the ZES, PPIs require dose escalation in only ~10% of ZES patients. Surgical tumor excision of the gastrinoma depends on a number of factors, and although the goal of definitive treatment, is beyond the scope of this discussion.

Upper GI hemorrhage (Table 2.4)

The role of acid suppression in the management of upper GI hemorrhage has been assessed in numerous studies, and no agent has proven to be unequivocally beneficial in patients without a specific diagnosis. On the other hand, several studies have shown a beneficial effect of antisecretory therapy in ulcer-related bleeding. The role of acid suppression alone,

Table 2.4 Treatment of bleeding peptic ulcers*

Proton pump inhibitor	Dose (adult) intravenous route
Pantoprazole, Omeprazole, Esomeprazole	80 mg bolus followed by 8 mg/hour**

*In general, patients with suspected significant upper GI bleeding should be started on high-dose IV PPI prior to endoscopy. Those patients without active bleeding or high risk stigmata of recent bleeding (visible vessel or adherent clot) can be switched to standard dose PPI therapy after endoscopy.
**Recommended duration of treatment is 72 hours for those patients with high-risk stigmata or active bleeding found on endoscopy before switching to oral therapy.

without endoscopic therapy, in the management of bleeding peptic ulcer, however, remains undefined. Only one study in which orally administered PPIs had been used demonstrated a significant reduction in the rate of recurrent bleeding in ulcers harboring nonbleeding visible vessels or a clot. This trend was not evident among those actively bleeding, suggesting that acid suppression with an oral PPI alone might stabilize clots.

A large study from Hong Kong compared combined endoscopic treatment and adjunct use of omeprazole infusion (80 mg loading dose, followed by an infusion of 8 mg/h) to the use of omeprazole infusion alone in the treatment of ulcers with nonbleeding visible vessels or clots. In those assigned to the combined treatment, recurrent bleeding occurred in 1 of 70 patients, on day 14 of treatment. In those patients receiving intravenous PPI infusion alone, the rate of recurrent bleeding was 11% at day 30. While the results clearly showed that combined therapy was superior in the control of bleeding, the low rate of recurrent bleeding in the PPI infusion alone group suggests that acid suppression does have a therapeutic role in ulcers with high-risk stigmata of recent hemorrhage (i.e., nonbleeding visible vessel and clot).

A systematic review of 9 trials (1829 patients) with either placebo or H2RAs as control revealed that PPI use correlated with reductions (OR 0.50, 95% CI 0.33 to 0.77; p = 0.002) in the rate of recurrent bleeding and need for surgery (OR 0.47, 95% CI 0.29 to 0.77; p = 0.003). The use of PPIs also led to an 8% (p=NS) reduction in the odds ratio for death. These findings suggest that PPIs are of benefit in the management of bleeding peptic ulcer. Importantly, no study to date has compared high-dose PPI infusion to an oral PPI after endoscopic hemostasis; thus there are no clear evidence-based guidelines regarding optimal route of dosing following endoscopic hemostasis. Intragastric pH control with oral PPI is suboptimal since the oral absorption of a PPI is not always reliable in critically ill patients. Based on the above studies, it would appear that the optimal approach to the management of bleeding peptic ulcer should include early endoscopic treatment for patients with high-risk ulcers, followed by a high-dose PPI infusion, as above, to prevent recurrent bleeding.

Stress ulcer bleeding

Stress-related lesions in the stomach and duodenum can be detected endoscopically within several hours of a critical illness, trauma, or surgery as multiple punctate subepithelial hemorrhages, erosions, or superficial ulcerations. Mucosal injury may be identified in 70–100% of critically ill patients admitted to an intensive care unit (ICU), and the risk of developing these lesions is directly correlated with the severity of the underlying illness. Most patients in an ICU are at risk for stress ulcer syndrome (SUS), and those with severe systemic disease represent the highest risk group. Mechanical ventilation for at least 48 hours and coagulopathy (platelet count of < 50 000, a partial thromboplastin time of more than twice that of control subjects, or an International Normalized Ratio of prothrombin time of > 1.5) have been identified as the two single most important risk factors.

Prophylactic therapy with H2RAs or with PPIs to inhibit gastric acid secretion has been used clinically to reduce the incidence of bleeding in SUS. However, a reduction in mortality due to bleeding remains unproven. No large randomized trials have been performed to date to evaluate the benefit of these agents in the prophylaxis of SUS-associated GI bleeding, although small studies suggest a beneficial effect. The rationale for this approach stems from *in vitro* studies where an increase of intragastric pH to 3.5 to 4.0 correlates with decreased conversion of pepsinogen to pepsin and reduced proteolytic activity in the stomach. Moreover, when intragastric pH approaches 7.0, pepsinogen is irreversibly denatured and clotting factors become operable, enabling activation of the coagulation cascade. Finally, platelet aggregation, which occurs only at a pH > 5.9, also contributes to successful hemostasis and prevention of bleeding due to SUS.

Studies comparing the ability of IV administrations of H2RAs and PPIs to increase and maintain intragastric pH suggest that, although both can raise the pH to > 4, PPIs are much more likely to maintain this pH. Unlike H2RAs, PPIs can elevate and maintain the intragastric pH at > 6, and unlike H2RAs, tolerance does not develop with IV preparations. Clinical trials conducted within an ICU setting have shown that intermittent administration of IV pantoprazole is as effective in raising intragastric pH on the first day as a continuous infusion of an H2RA. These data suggest that intermittent or continuous infusion with an IV PPI may be an alternative to high-dose continuous infusions of an H2RA. If continuous

IV infusion is used, the recommended dose of a PPI is an 80 mg loading dose, followed by an infusion of 8 mg/h.

Difficulties in the nasogastric/orogastric (NG/OG) tube administration of omeprazole and lansoprazole to mechanically ventilated ICU patients have not been resolved despite the recent development of suspensions that are somewhat effective in keeping gastric pH >4. Two studies in mechanically ventilated ICU patients suggested that Zegurid® (omeprazole in bicarbonate solution) might not only prevent clinically significant SRES-related hemorrhage, but is also safe and cost-effective. However, omeprazole and lansoprazole have been formulated as granules with an enteric coating designed to dissolve at pH 5.5, but are still acid labile prodrugs. Thus, the protective enteric coating may be dissolved within the highly alkaline bicarbonate suspension. Although the drug is purportedly protected from the acidic environment in the gastric lumen by the bicarbonate, many other factors may influence acid exposure, including the amount of bicarbonate, as well as the pH and volume of the solution used to flush the suspension through a nasogastric tube. Unfortunately, it is still possible that the PPI released from the granules undergoes acid-catalyzed conversion to its thiophilic sulfenamide, with inactivation of the drug before arrival at its intended target site.

Nonulcer dyspepsia

Dyspepsia is a common symptom, occurring in up to 40% of the population. And, of those patients seeking medical care, dyspepsia accounts for roughly 5% of primary care office visits. In the United States, the point prevalence approximates 25% once patients with typical reflux symptoms are excluded. The best approach to the patient with uninvestigated dyspepsia remains a topic of debate, a debate initially fueled by the uncertain appropriateness of empirical treatment without endoscopic evaluation in conjunction with a strong desire for cost containment. The evaluation of dyspepsia is beyond the scope of this chapter. Nonulcer dyspepsia, also known as functional or idiopathic dyspepsia, is defined as the presence of one or more of the following symptoms (epigastric burning/fullness, postprandial fullness, early satiation), without a structural or organic etiology after a negative diagnostic evaluation.

Although nonulcer dyspepsia comprises many disease entities, a 4-8 week treatment course with a PPI is effective for many patients with dyspepsia and an acceptable initial management approach for patients without alarm features, many of whom will never need investigation. PPIs have supplanted H2RAs in this cost-containing approach, and prokinetic agents with established efficacy in this role presently are unavailable in the United States. Risks of empirical antisecretory treatment primarily include under-treatment and failing to diagnose a serious medical condition, such as malignancy. The diagnosis of ulcer disease could be established with endoscopy at relapse, and, in fact, most of the diagnoses responsible for dyspepsia persist or relapse after discontinuation of therapy. Relapse with functional dyspepsia can be expected in at least two-thirds of patients in relatively short follow-up. The high relapse rates of the common causes for dyspepsia result in most patients undergoing endoscopy within one year, thus reducing the risks associated with empirical antisecretory treatment.

Adverse effects/safety

Common side effects of PPIs include headache, abdominal pain, nausea, vomiting, diarrhea and constipation, which ranges from 1-10%. Serious adverse reactions are rare. As mentioned above, with the exception of omeprazole, which is listed as pregnancy category C due to adverse events reported in animal reproduction studies, all other PPIs are listed as pregnancy category B.

Long-term maintenance therapy use of PPIs in conditions such as GERD has raised specific concerns of chronic acid suppression resulting in prolonged hypochlorhydria, hypergastrinemia and possibly atrophic gastritis. Although there have been concerns regarding the theoretical risk of developing carcinomas or carcinoid tumors due to hypergastrinemia and chronic atrophic gastritis, no clear causality has been established in humans with use of PPIs. The safety concerns with hypochlorhydria include potential increased risk for infection and malabsorption. There is potential for increased risk of infections, specifically enteric infections, *Clostridium difficile*-Associated Diarrhea (CDAD), and community acquired pneumonia (CAP). Although patients who developed CDAD had other potential risk factors, association with PPI use could not be ruled out; thus, the US Food and Drug Administration (FDA) issued a special alert to providers to consider the diagnosis if patients have symptoms that could be consistent with CDAD, and to use the lowest possible dose and shortest duration of PPI therapy appropriate for the condition.

PPIs have also been associated with a 1.27 fold increase in the risk of community acquired pneumonia in a meta-analysis of observational studies. The precise mechanism is not known, but is thought to be possibly due to hypochlorhydria, allowing a permissive environment for bacterial pathogens. Another study challenges that this association may be confounded, as the authors were able to correlate PPI use with other medical conditions that did not seem to have a plausible biological explanation or mechanism. For those patients on chronic PPI therapy, decreased absorption of magnesium, calcium, iron and vitamin B12 have been potential concerns. Recommendations to clinicians include periodic monitoring and/or supplementation. Results of the Women's Health Initiative demonstrated a slightly increased risk between 1.25 fold for total fractures (spine, forearm, wrist, hip) in postmenopausal women on PPIs, but no significant difference at 3 years on bone mineral density measurements.

Chronic, long-term use of PPIs of more than 12 months has been associated with development of fundic gland polyps, though the mechanism is not fully understood. Regression of these benign polyps has also been described after PPI withdrawal. Apart from those patients with familial adenomatous polyposis, these polyps do not require removal or surveillance. There is also ongoing debate on whether PPIs, specifically lansoprazole, is associated with the development of microscopic colitis, with some studies showing clinical improvement when changing to another PPI and other studies showing no increased association with PPIs.

As mentioned previously, PPIs should not be given *concomitantly* with other antisecretory agents such as H2RAs, because of the marked reduction in acid inhibitory effect. H2RAs can be used with PPIs but need to be administered sequentially several hours apart.

Although studies have shown that concomitant use of clopidogrel and PPI, specifically omeprazole, reduces the antiplatelet effect of clopidogrel, it has not been clearly established whether this observation translates into a clinically important interaction regarding cardiovascular risk. Hypothetical PPI-antiplatelet interactions include competitive inhibition of CYP2C19 by PPIs or genetic polymorphisms in the hepatic cytochrome P450 family of enzymes, but the exact mechanism is unknown. In general, PPIs are appropriate to use in patients with multiple risk factors for GI bleeding who require anti platelet therapy. Overall, a multi-society taskforce of cardiologists and gastroenterologists recommends that clinical decisions regarding concomitant use of PPIs with thienopyridines must be guided by overall risks and benefits of cardiovascular and GI complications.

PPIs may decrease the serum concentration of some drugs and should not be given concomitantly with: dasatinib (chemotherapeutic agent), pimozide (antipsychotic used to treat Tourette's syndrome), posaconzale (antifungal), delayed release risendronate (bisphosphonate), and delavirdine (antiretroviral agent used to treat HIV). The herbal St. John's Wort may decrease the concentration of omeprazole and should be avoided in combination.

Recommended reading

ACCF/ACG/AHA (2010) Expert Consensus Document on the Concomitant Use of Proton Pump Inhibitors and Thienopyridines: A focused update of the ACCF/ACG/AHA 2008 Expert Consensus Document on Reducing the Gastrointestinal Risks of Antiplatelet Therapy and NSAID Use. *Am J Gastroenterol* **105**: 2533–49.

Barrison AF, Jarboe LA, Weinberg BM, Nimmagadda K, Sullivan LM, Wolfe, MM (2001) Patterns of proton pump inhibitor use in clinical practice. *Am J Med* **111**: 469–73.

Bavishi C, Dupont HL (2011) Systematic review: the use of proton pump inhibitors and increased susceptibility to enteric infection. *Aliment Pharmacol Ther* **34**: 1269–81.

Cook DJ, Fuller HD, Guyatt GH, *et al.* (1994) Risk factors for gastrointestinal bleeding in critically ill patients. Canadian Critical Care Trials Group. *N Engl J Med* **330**: 377–81.

Dial, MS (2009) Proton pump inhibitor use and enteric infections. *Am J Gastroenterol* **104**: S10–S16.

Eom CS, Jeon CY, Lim JW *et al.* (2011) Use of acid-suppressive drugs and risk of pneumonia: a systematic review and meta-analysis. *CMAJ* **183**: 310–19.

Fellenius E, Berglindh T, Sachs G *et al.* (1981) Substituted benzimidazoles inhibit gastric acid secretion by blocking (H+, K+) ATPase. *Nature* **290**: 159–61.
In this paper, the authors isolated and characterized the substituted benzimidazole, which they found inhibited the hydrogen potassium ATPase, the final step in acid secretion in the parietal cell. This discovery is the foundation for the development of modern class of proton pump inhibitors.

Gray SL, LaCroix AZ, Larson J, *et al.* (2010) Proton pump inhibitor use, hip fracture, and change in bone mineral density in post menopausal women: results from the women's health initiative. *Arch Intern Med* **170**: 765–71.

Guiliano C, Wilhem SM, Kale-Pradhan PB (2012) Are proton pump inhibitors associated with the development of community acquired pneumonia? A meta-analysis. *Expert Rev Clin Pharmacol* **5**: 337–44.

Insogna KL (2009) The effect of proton pump inhibiting drugs on mineral metabolism. *Am J Gastroenterol* **104**: S2–S4.

Janarthanan S, Ditah I, Adler DG, Ehrinpreis MN (2012) *Clostridium difficile* associated diarrhea and proton pump inhibitor therapy: a meta analysis. *Am J Gastroenterol* **107**: 1001–10.

Jena AB, Sun E, Goldman DP (2012) Confounding in the Association of proton pump inhibitor use with risk of community acquired pneumonia. *J Gen Intern Med* **28**: 223–30.

Lodato, F, Azzaroli F, Turco L, Mazzella N, Buonfiglioli F, Zoli M, Mazzella, G (2010) Adverse effects of proton pump inhibitors. *Best Pract and Res Clinical Gastroenterol* **24**: 193–201.

Metz DC, Soffer E, Forsmark CE, *et al.* Maintenance oral pantoprazole therapy is effective for patients with Zollinger-Ellison Syndrome and idiopathic hypersecretion. *Am J Gastroenterol* 2003;**98**:301–7.

Oviedo JA, Wolfe MM (2005) Management of stress related erosive syndrome. In TM Bayless, A Diehl (eds), *Advanced Therapy in Gastroenterology and Liver Disease*. Michigan: BC Decker, pp. 161–6.

Scheiman JM, Yeomans ND, Talley NJ, Vakil N, Chan FK, Tulassay Z, Rainoldi JL, Szczepanski L, Ung KA, Kleczkowski D, Ahlbom H, Naesdal J, Hawkey C (2006) Prevention of ulcers by esomeprazole in at-risk patients using non-selective NSAIDs and COX-2 inhibitors. *Am J Gastroenterol* **101**: 701–10.

Scheiman JM, Devereaux PJ, Herlitz J, Katelaris PH, Lanas A, Veldhuyzen van Zanten S, Nauclér E, Svedberg LE (2011) Prevention of peptic ulcers with esomeprazole in patients at risk of ulcer development treated with low dose acetylsalicylic acid: a randomized, controlled trial (OBERON). *Heart* **97**: 797–802.

Singh G, Triadafilodopoulos G (2005) Appropriate choice of proton pump inhibitor therapy in the prevention and management of NSAID-related gastrointestinal damage. *Internat J Clin Prac* **59**: 1210–17.

Wolfe MM, Sachs G (2000) Acid suppression: optimizing therapy for gastroduodenal healing, gastroesophageal reflux disease, and stress related erosive syndrome. *Gastroenterology* **118**: S9–S31.

The authors review the pathophysiology of acid secretion and acid related disorders, pharmacology of drugs used to treat these disorders, and safety issues related to medications. A comprehensive review targeted for the clinician.

Wolfe MM, Soll AH (1988) The physiology of gastric acid secretion. *N Engl J Med* **319**: 1707–15.

Wolfe MM, Lichtenstein DR, Singh G (1999) Gastrointestinal toxicity of nonsteroidal antiinflammatory drugs. *N Engl J Med* **340**: 1888–99.

An excellent review of the epidemiology, pathogenesis, prevention and treatment of NSAID related gastroduodenal mucosal injury, it has been cited by over 100 publications, and remains an important review article.

Wolfe MM, Welage LS, Sachs G (2001) Proton pump inhibitors and gastric acid secretion. *Am J Gastroenterol* **96**: 3467–8.

Yang Y, Metz D (2010) Safety of proton pump inhibitor exposure. *Gastroenterology* **139**: 1115–27.

A comprehensive review of the pathophysiology and safety profile of PPIs with detailed discussion regarding mechanism of action of PPIs, summary of adverse effects of PPI therapy and provide clinicians with guidelines to minimize potential for adverse outcomes of treatment.

CHAPTER 3

Histamine H$_2$-receptor antagonists

Kentaro Sugano
Jichi Medical University, Shimotsuke, Tochigi, Japan

Introduction

Drug development targeting human histamine receptors have been rewarded with the successful launching of H$_1$- and H$_2$-receptor antagonists in clinical use. Currently, two additional histamine receptors (H$_3$ and H$_4$) have been identified, for which intensive efforts have been made for developing new drugs (Table 3.1). These new antihistamine H$_3$- and H$_4$-receptor antagonists are aimed at treating allergic diseases (asthma, allergic rhinitis) or disorders affecting the central nervous system (Alzheimer's disease, narcolepsy) and are still in their clinical development stages. Because their application in digestive diseases remains uncertain, this chapter will focus on H$_2$-receptor antagonists and their clinical pharmacology.

Mechanism of action

Histamine has been recognized as a potent stimulant of acid secretion, but conventional antihistamine (H$_1$) compounds used to treat allergic conditions generally possessed poor inhibitory capacity in terms of acid suppression. Therefore, the presence of a separate class of histamine receptor responsible for acid secretion was predicted and, as a result, intensive efforts for drug development were pursued. In the early 1970s metiamide, the first compound specific to the H$_2$ receptor, was evaluated for the treatment of peptic ulcer diseases and demonstrated superior effects over a placebo in terms of symptomatic relief and ulcer healing. Unfortunately, metiamide was withdrawn early due to bone marrow toxicity, which occurred as a result of its thiourea group. Subsequently, however, with the replacement of the thiourea for a cyanoguanidine group, cimetidine was introduced into clinical use. It revolutionized the management of peptic ulcer diseases with dramatically improved effects on

Pocket Guide to Gastrointestinal Drugs, Edited by M. Michael Wolfe and Robert C. Lowe. © 2014
John Wiley & Sons, Ltd. Published 2014 by John Wiley & Sons, Ltd.

Table 3.1 Human histamine receptors

Subtype	Chromosome	Signal transduction	Tissue distribution	Physiological function
H_1	3p25	Gq/G_{11}	Heart, brain, mast cells	Modulation of smooth muscle contraction, Modulation of neurotransmission, Vasodilation
H_2	5q35.2	Gq/G_{11}, Gs	Heart, brain, neutrophil, parietal cells	Stimulation of gastric acid Modulation of leucocyte function
H_3	20q13.33	Gi/G_0	Brain, peripheral nervous system	Modulation of central nervous system activity
H_4	18q11.2	Gi/G_0	Blood cells (mast cells, eosinophils, monocytes)	Modulation of allergic reaction Gi/G_0

Four subtypes of human histamine receptors with distinct tissue distribution and physiological functions are currently known. Drug development for histamine receptor antagonists for newer subtypes are ongoing.

symptomatic control, as well as ulcer healing, compared to conventional treatment with antacids and anticholinergic drugs.

Following the brilliant success of cimetidine, many drugs acting as H_2-receptor specific antagonists (H2RAs), such as ranitidine, famotidine, and nizatidine, have been developed and marketed all over the world. Two more H2RAs, roxatidine acetate and lafutidine, are also available in Japan and other Asian countries (Figure 3.1).

These compounds bind to histamine H_2 receptors on parietal cells (see Chapter 2, Figure 2.2) and thereby antagonize the action of histamine. In addition, some of these H2RAs have other actions unique to each compound, such as immune modulation by cimetidine, stimulation of salivary secretion by nizatidine, and stimulation of gastric mucus secretion by roxatidine and lafutidine.

Although histamine is the major activation signal for stimulating acid secretion, other secretagogues, such as cholinergic stimulation or gastrin, can also stimulate acid secretion independent from histamine. Therefore,

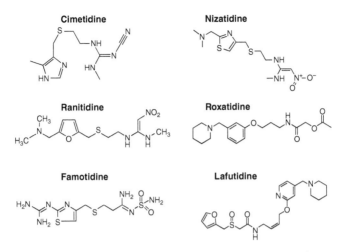

Figure 3.1 Chemical structure of histamine H$_2$-receptor antagonists.

acid inhibition by H2RAs is less potent compared to proton pump inhibitors (PPIs) that target H$^+$, K$^+$-ATPase, which is the final common enzyme responsible for acid secretion activated by all secretagogues.

Pharmacology

Most H2RAs developed early have imidazole (cimetidine), furan (ranitidine), or thiazole (famotidine and nizatidine) structures that simulate the imidazole ring of histamine as their chemical backbones. Newly introduced H2RAs, such as roxatidine acetate and lafutidine, however, have different chemical structures (Figure 3.1). All of these drugs are administered orally, but parenteral preparations are also available for most of these drugs. The absorption of H2RAs is rapid and reaches peak concentration in 1–3 hours. They all show good bioavailability, ranging from 30 to 100%.

Regular doses for healing peptic ulcers are quite different (Table 3.2), which reflects their relative potencies with regard to acid inhibition. Although once daily regimens are effective in healing ulcers, especially when given at bedtime, they are commonly given in two divided doses because of their short serum half-lives (1–4 hours). In general, H2RAs are metabolized in the liver, but renal excretion also contributes to their elimination. There are considerable differences in the relative contributions of hepatic and renal pathway for each drug. For nizatidine, the kidney plays a major role in elimination, whereas heaptic metabolism contributes more to the disposition of cimetidine, ranitidine, and famotidine.

Table 3.2 Histamine H_2-receptor antagonists

Compound	Trade names (USA/EU/Japan) *	Indications	Regular dose (Adult)	Parenteral dose	Pregnancy Category (FDA)	Important Drug Interactions[#]
Cimetidine	Tagamet® (USA/EU/Japan)	Active peptic ulcer (GU/DU),	USA: 800 mg~1600 mg hs, 400 mg bid, 300 mg qid Japan: 400 mg bid or 200 mg qid	USA: 300 mg iv or im every 6 to 8 hrs or 37.5~50 mg/hr drip infusion	B	cisapride clopidogrel
		USA: Prophylaxis for DU	USA:400 mg hs	USA: 300 mg iv or im 1 or 2/day		carmustine
		Zollinger-Ellison syndrome	USA: 300 mg qid, Japan:200 mg qid or 400 mg bid	USA: 300 mg iv or im every 6 hrs or 40~600 mg/hr drip infusion (Max 2.4 g/d)		epirubicin
		Reflux Esophagitis	USA: 800 m bid, 400 mg qid Japan: 400 mg bid, or 200 mg qid	USA: 300 mg iv or im equiv 6 hr, or 50 mg/hr drip infusion (Max 2.4g/d)		phenytoin pimozide
		Gastritis or Dyspepsia	200 mg bid			phenytoin
		Premedication before general anesthesia		Japan: 200 mg im before anesthesia		tamoxifen
		UGI bleeding (PUB, hemorrhagic gastritis)		USA: 150 mg bolus iv followed by 50 mg/hr di (Max:2.4 g/d) Japan: 200 mg iv or di, q6 hr		theophylline warfarin

Ranitidine hydrochloride	Zantac® (USA/EU Japan)			B	
	Active peptic ulcer (GU/DU),	150 mg bid or 300 mg hs	50 mg iv or im every 6-8 hrs, or 6.25mg/kg/hr drip infusion		gefitinib
	USA: Prophylaxis for DU,	150 mg hs			metophormin
	USA: Maintenance for GU	150 mg hs			pheynytoin
	Zollinger-Ellison syndrome	USA: 150 mg bid (USA: increase the dose up to 6 g/d), Japan 150 mg bid	USA: 1 mg/kg/hr drip infusion (max 2.5mg/kg/hr)		theophylline
	USA: Hypersecretory conditions	USA: 150 mg bid (USA: increase the dose up to 6 g/d)			triazolam
	Reflux Esophagitis	150 mg bid	50 mg iv or im every 6-8 hrs, or 6.25mg/kg/hr drip infusion		warfarin
	Gastritis or Dyspepsia	USA: 75 mg hs or 75 mg bid, Japan 150 mg hs, or 75 mg bid			
	Premedication before general anesthesia		50 mg im or iv before anesthesia		
	UGI bleeding (PUB, hemorrhagic gastritis)		USA: 50 mg iv loading followed by 6.25 mg/hr drip infusion Japan: 50 mg 3-4× iv/d or 100 mg 2x drip infusion/d		

(continued)

Table 3.2 (*Continued*)

Compound	Trade names (USA/EU/Japan) *	Indications	Regular dose (Adult)	Parenteral dose	Pregnancy Category (FDA)	Important Drug Interactions#
Famotidine	Pepcid® (USA/ EU)/Gaster® (Japan)	Active peptic ulcer (GU/DU),	40 mg hs or 20 mg bid	USA: 20 mg iv every 12 hrs	B	gefitinib
		Prophylaxis of DU	20 mg sid	USA: 20 mg iv once/d		ketoconazole
		Zollinger-Ellison syndrome	USA: 20 mg every 6 hrs (up to 160 mg every 6 hrs), Japan: 20 mg bid, 40 mg hs	USA 20 mg iv every 6 hrs		phenytoin
		USA: Hypersecretory conditions	USA: 20 mg every 6 hrs (up to 160 mg every 6 hrs)	USA: 20 mg iv every 6 hrs		theophylline
		Reflux Esophagitis	USA: 20 to 40 mg bid, Japan: 20 mg bid or 40 mg hs	USA: 20 mg iv every 12 hrs		tizanidine
		Gastritis or Dyspepsia	USA: 10 mg sid or bid, Japan: 10 mg bid			
		Premedication before general anesthesia		Japan:20 mg iv 2x/d		
		UGI bleeding (PUB, hemorrhagic gastritis)		20 mg iv 2x/d		

Drug	Brands	Indication	Dose		Category	Interactions
Nizatidine	Axid® (USA)/ Axid®, Tazac® (EU)/Acinon® (Japan)	Peptic ulcer (GU/DU),	150 mg bid or 300 mg hs	NA	B	atazanavir, gefitinib, ketoconazole, phenytoin, prulifloxacin, theophyliline
		Reflux Esophagitis	150 mg bid			
		Gastritis or Dyspepsia	75 mg hs or bid, Japan: 75 mg bid			
Roxatidine acetate hydrochloride	NA/NA/Altat®	Peptic ulcer (GU/DU)	Japan: 75 mg bid,150 mg hs		C	
		Zollinger-Ellison syndrome	Japan: 75 mg bid			
		Reflux Esophagitis	Japan: 75 mg bid,150 mg hs			
		Gastritis	Japan: 75 mg hs			
		Premedication before general anesthesia	Japan: 75 mg bid,150 mg hs before anesthesia	Japan: 75mg iv before anesthesia		
		UGI bleeding (PUB, AGML)		Japan 75mg di 2x iv/d		
2368	NA/NA/ Protecadin®, Stoger®	Peptic ulcer (GU/DU),	Japan: 10 mg bid	NA	C	
		Reflux Esophagitis	Japan: 10 mg bid			
		Gastritis	Japan: 10 mg sid			

Table 3.2 (Continued)

Compound	Trade names (USA/EU/Japan) *	Indications	Regular dose (Adult)	Parenteral dose	Pregnancy Category (FDA)	Important Drug Interactions#
Famotidine/ anti-acid famotidine (10 mg)/calcium carbonate (800 mg)/ magnesium hydroxide (165 mg)	Pepcid Complete® (USA)/ Pepcidduo®, Pepciddual® Pepcidtwo®, Pepcid Duo® (EU)/NA (Japan)	Heartburn	USA: prn	NA	B	See famotidine
Ranitidine bismuth citrate (Ranitidine 162 mg + trivalent bismuth 128 mg + 110 mg citrate)	NA (USA)/ Tritec® (EU)/ NA (Japan)	Eradication therapy for *Helicobacter pylori*	400 mg bid with clarithromycin	NA	C	See ranitidine

(continued)

Famotidine/ Ibuprofen (famotidine 26.6 mg, ibuprofen 800 mg)	Duexis® (USA)/ NA/NA	osteoarthritis and rheumatoid arthritis	tid	NA	C	See famotidine

NA: not available

* See more detailed information on Drugs.Com (http://www.drugs.com/)

\# See more detailed infromation on Drugs. Com (http://www.drugs.com/drug_interactions.html)

Histamine H2 receptor antagonists (H2RAs) used in the global market. Some of them are not available in the USA. Most of the H2RAs are available as generics and over-the counter drugs with variety of brand names. Numerous brand names are registered for cimetidine, ranitidine, famotidine, nizatidine, and roxatidine in each country. H2RAs in combination with other drugs are also commercialized.

Websites listing additional brand names for histamine H2-receptor antagonists:

Cimetidine: http://www.drugs.com/international/cimetidine.html
Ranitidine: http://www.bddrugs.com/product5.php?idn=3
Famotidine: http://www.egeneralmedical.com/rxlist00000301.html
Nizatidine: http://www.drugs.com/international/nizatidine.html
Roxatidine: http://www.drugs.com/international/roxatidine.html
Lafutidine: http://www.drugs.com/international/lafutidine.html

Notably, cimetidine is mostly metabolized through cytochrome enzymes, including CYP2C9 and CYP3A4, which are responsible for metabolizing many other drugs, such as warfarin, and consideration should thus be given when co-prescribing drugs that share the same metabolic disposition pathways. Nevertheless, all these H2RAs require dose reductions when renal function is impaired. The only exception is lafutidine, which undergoes hepatic metabolism, with the majority of the metabolites being excreted into stool.

Currently available H2RAs should be classified pharmacologically as inverse agonists rather than true antagonists. The sustained use of H2RAs stimulates up-regulation of H_2 receptors, which may explain tolerance and a rebound phenomenon that may occur upon cessation of H2RA therapy.

Clinical effectiveness

Since H2RAs exert their properties by suppressing acid secretion, their main clinical application is the treatment of acid-related diseases, such as peptic ulcer diseases, gastroesophageal reflux disease (GERD), and erosive gastritis. Ulcer healing rates associated with H2RAs usually averages approximately 80% for duodenal ulcer in 4 weeks and gastric ulcer in 8 weeks. However, H2RAs have not been proven effective in the treatment of GI hemorrhage due to peptic ulceration; and endoscopic hemostasis, combined with PPI, remains the treatment of choice (see Chapter 2). H2RAs are also used for preventing stress-related ulcers and secondary hemorrhagic events before surgery and for patients with severe burns ("Curling's" ulcers) and head injury ("Cushing's" ulcers). Some studies have also shown H2RAs to be effective in reducing nonsteroidal anti-inflammatory drug (NSAID)-induced duodenal ulcer, and to a lesser extent gastric ulcer, as well as in low-dose aspirin (LDA) induced ulcer. Recently a single-tablet combination of ibuprofen and high-dose famotidine was introduced into market. However, the beneficial properties of H2RAs on clinically relevant indices, including upper GI bleeding associated with the use of NSAID or LDA are inferior to PPIs (see Chapter 2), and the use of H2RAs is thus not recommended for high-risk group patients. For patients receiving clopidogrel therapy, however, H2RAs may offer protection and benefit because of the possibility of an interaction of PPIs on the activation of clopidogrel through CYP2C19.

H2RAs are effective in achieving symptomatic relief and healing of erosive GERD, but the overall efficacy in symptomatic relief and healing rates for esophageal mucosal injury is less satisfactory when compared with PPIs. In particular, high grade esophagitis is resistant or refractory to H2RAs and requires more potent and prolonged acid inhibition with

PPIs. For patients with nocturnal acid breakthrough (NAB), the bedtime administration of H2RA was advocated to enhance acid inhibition during the night when PPI action may be inadequate. However, it was subsequently shown that the beneficial effects of H2RA on NAB were transient, thus lessening enthusiasm for long-term use with these agents. H2RAs alone or in combination with an antacid regimen may be used for the symptomatic control of heartburn and/or dyspepsia.

For the treatment of the Zollinger-Ellison syndrome (ZES), a high initial dose of H2RAs is necessary for controlling basal acid secretion (<10 mmol/hour), and further dose escalations are usually necessary to maintain their antisecretory effects. PPIs are far more effective in inhibiting acid secretion, and these agents are accordingly the mainstay of therapy in this disease entity (see Chapter 2).

Although H2RAs are rarely used for the eradication therapy of *Helicobacter pylori*, the superiority of PPI-based therapy over H2RA-based regimens is somewhat controversial. Direct comparative studies with lafutidine-based triple therapy and lansoprazole-based triple therapy were shown to exhibit equal eradication rate. Moreover, ranitidine-bismuth has been used as a key component of eradication regimen where available.

Adverse events

H2RAs are well known for their proven safety profile. However, they have been associated with adverse events, such as bone marrow suppression, liver injury, interstitial nephritis, and dysfunction of the central nervous system (CNS). Elderly people are more susceptible to CNS dysfunction, including agitation, mental confusion, delirium, and psychosis. In addition to drug interactions through drug metabolizing enzymes, other interactions also occur. For example, due to acid suppression by H2RA, the absorption of certain drugs, such as ketoconazole and gefitinib, can be reduced, thereby necessitating dose- adjustment.

It is also known that the sudden cessation of H2RAs can precipitate in a "rebound phenomenon" in which acid secretion increases after the discontinuation of H2RAs, likely occurring as a result of inverse agonism properties of H2RA. Clinically, this phenomenon may lead relapse of peptic ulcers, and therefore, a 50% dose reduction of H2RAs is often maintained for a prolonged period to reduce ulcer recurrence (maintenance therapy). In the era of eradication therapy, however, maintenance therapy is far less frequently employed after the successful eradication of *H. pylori*, but maintenance therapy may be indicated for *H. pylori*-negative ulcer patients with ulcer recurrences.

Most H2RAs are pregnancy category B, but H2RAs may be transmitted by lactating mothers. Because the concentration of cimetidine and ranitidine in breast milk is much higher than circulating concentrations, famotidine may be preferred in this situation because of lesser gradient.

Recommended reading

Abraham NS, Hlatky MA, Antman EM, *et al.* (2010) ACCF/ACG/AHA 2010 expert consensus document on the concomitant use of proton pump inhibitors and thienopyridines; a focused update of the ACCF/ACG/AHA 2008 expert consensus documents on reducing the gastrointestinal risks of antiplatelet therapy and NSAID use. *Am J Gastroenterol* **105**: 2533–49.
Guidelines formulated by a multi-society task force and are the current standard for preventing gastrointestinal injury associated with the use of nonsteroidal anti-inflammatory drugs and anti-platelet agents.

Barkun AN, Cockeram AW, Plourde V, *et al.* (1999) Review article: acid suppression in non-variceal acute upper gastrointestinal bleeding. *Aliment Pharmacol Ther* **13**: 1565–84.

Cantu TG, Korek JS (1991) Central nervous system reactions to histamine-2 receptor blockers. *Ann Intern Med* **114**: 1027–34.

Chan FK, Abraham NS, Scheiman JM, *et al.* (2008) Management of patients on nonsteroidal anti-inflammatory drugs: a clinical practice recommendation from the First International Working Party on Gastrointestinal and Cardiovascular Effects of Nonsteroidal Anti-inflammatory Drugs and Anti-platelet Agents. *Am J Gastroenterol* **103**: 2008–18.

Chiba N, De Gara CJ, Wilkinson JM, *et al.* (1997) Speed of healing and symptom relief in Grade II to IV gastroesophageal reflux disease: A meta-analysis. *Gastroenterology* **112**: 1798–1810.

Fackler WK, Ours TM, Vaezi MF, *et al.* (2002) Long-term effect of H2RA therapy on nocturnal gastric acid breakthrough. *Gastroenterology* **122**: 625–32.

Feldman M, Burton ME (1990a) Histamine2-receptor antagonists. Standard therapy for acid-peptic diseases (first of two parts). *N Engl J Med* **323**: 1672–80.

Feldman M, Burton ME (1990b) Histamine2-receptor antagonists. Standard therapy for acid-peptic diseases (second of two parts). *N Engl J Med* **323**; 1749–55
Most comprehensive reviews on H2RA published in two separate issues.

Gisbert JP, Khorrami S, Calvet X, *et al.* Meta-analysis: proton pump inhibitors vs. H2-receptor antagonists: their efficacy with antibiotics in *Helicobacter pylori* eradication. *Aliment Pharmacol Ther* **18**: 757–66.

Gisbert JP, Gonzalez L, Calvet X (2005) Systematic review and meta-analysis: proton pump inhibitor vs. ranitidine bismuth citrate plus two antibiotics in *Helicobacter pylori* eradication. *Helicobacter* **10**: 157–71.

Graham DY, Hammoud F, El-Zemaity HMT, *et al.* Meta-analysis: proton pump inhibitor or H2-receptor antagonist for *Helicobacter pylori* eradication. *Aliment Pharmacol Ther* **17**: 1229.

Hill SJ, Chazot P, Fukui H, *et al.* (n.d.) http://www.iuphar-db.org/DATABASE/FamilyMenuForward?familyId=33 (accessed August 11, 2013).

Hudson N, Taha AS, Russell RI, *et al.* (1997) Famotidine for healing and maintenance in nonsteroidal anti-inflammatory drug-associated gastroduodenal ulceration. *Gastroenterology* **112**: 1817–22.

Isomoto H, Inoue K, Furusu H, *et al.* (2003) Lafutidine, a novel histamine H2-receptor antagonist, vs. lansoprazole in combination with amoxicillin and clarithromycin for eradication of *Helicobacter pylori*. *Helicobacter* **8**: 111–19

Laine L, Kivitz AJ, Bello AE, *et al.* (2012) Double-blind randomized trials of single-tablet ibuprofen/high-dose famotidine vs. ibuprofen alone for reduction of gastric and duodenal ulcers. *Am J Gastroenterol* **107**: 379–86.

Leurs R, Vischer HF, Wijtmans M, *et al.* (2011) En route to new blockbuster antihistamines: surveying the offspring of the expanding histamine receptor family. *Trends Pharmacol Sci* **32**: 250–7.
  Detailed review on current status of drug development on new histamine H$_3$ and H$_4$ antagonists.

Lin KJ, Hernandez-Diaz S, Garcia Rodriguez LA (2011) Acid suppressants reduce risk of gastrointestinal bleeding in patients on antithrombotic or anti-inflammatory therapy. *Gastroenterology* **141**: 71–9.

Maton PN, Vinayek R, Frucht H, *et al.* (1989) Long-term efficacy and safety of omeprazole in patients with Zollinger-Ellison syndrome: a prospective study. *Gastroenterology* **97**: 827–36

Nwokolo CU, Smith JT, Sawyer AM *et al.* (1991) Rebound intragastric hyperacidity after abrupt withdrawal of histamine H2 receptor blockade. *Gut* **32**: 1455–60.

Ren Q, Ma B, Yang K, *et al.* (2010) Lafutidine-based triple therapy for *Helicobacter pylori* eradication. *Hepatogastroenterology* **57**: 1074–81.

Richter JE (2005) Review article: the management of heartburn in pregnancy. *Aliment Pharmacol Ther* **22**: 749–57.

Smit MJ, Leurs R, Alewinese AE, *et al.* (1996) Inverse agonism of histamine H2 antagonists accounts for upregulation of spontaneously active histamine H2 receptors. *Proc Natl Acad Sci* **93**: 6802–7.

Taha AS McCloskey C, Prasad R, *et al.* (2009) Famotidine for the prevention of peptic ulcers and oesophagitis in patients taking low-dose aspirin (FAMOUS): a phase III, randomized, double-blind, placebo-controlled trial. *Lancet* **374**: 119–25.
  Good evidence for regular dose of famotidine in preventing upper gastrointestinal tract injury by low-dose aspirin is presented.

Wu CY, Chan FKL, Wu MS, *et al.* (2010) Histamine2-receptor antagonists are an alternative to proton pump inhibitor in patients receiving clopidogrel. *Gastroenterology* **139**: 1165–71.

CHAPTER 4

Prostaglandins and other mucosal protecting agents

Carlos Sostres and Angel Lanas
University Hospital, IIS Aragón, Zaragoza, Spain

Introduction of drug class

The history of prostaglandins began in the 1930s with the observation by two New York gynecologists, Kurzrok and Lieb, that human semen caused contractions and relaxation of human myometrium. These observations were soon confirmed by Goldblatt in England and by von Euler in Sweden. Indeed, these compounds were so named because they were believed (incorrectly) to be derived from prostatic secretions. A crucial discovery, in terms of understanding the role of prostaglandins in the stomach, was the finding by Vane in 1971 that aspirin, indomethacin, and other nonsteroidal anti-inflammatory drugs (NSAIDs) inhibited the synthesis of prostaglandins. Vane suggested that the inhibition of prostaglandin biosynthesis by NSAIDs may underlie the ability of this class of drugs to induce ulceration in the gastrointestinal tract. Vane also proposed that this mechanism accounted for the anti-inflammatory properties of these compounds, since prostaglandins were known at the time to contribute to edema formation and to the pain associated with inflammation.

In the decade that followed Vane's prediction, the phenomenon of "cytoprotection" was introduced into the literature by André Robert, who described the unexpected and fascinating finding that prostaglandins, the major metabolic products of arachidonic acid resulting from cyclooxygenase activity, can be crucial for the maintenance of gastroduodenal mucosal integrity. His group provided the experimental evidence that prostaglandins, when applied exogenously in nonantisecretory doses, exhibit high activity in preventing the mucosal damage induced by necrotizing substances, such as ethanol, hyperosmolar solutions, strong acids, alkaline substances, concentrated bile, and even

Pocket Guide to Gastrointestinal Drugs, Edited by M. Michael Wolfe and Robert C. Lowe. © 2014 John Wiley & Sons, Ltd. Published 2014 by John Wiley & Sons, Ltd.

boiling water. The precise mechanism of this so-called cytoprotective property of prostaglandins remained unknown, but the stimulatory effects of these agents on gastric mucus and bicarbonate secretions, an increase in the gastric microcirculation, and the enhancement in the mucosal sulfhydryl compounds were initially proposed to explain this phenomenon.

Prostaglandins were identified as a group of compounds rather than a single substance, and arachidonic acid was identified as their precursor. It was recognized that prostaglandins were produced by nearly all biologic tissues. Profound pharmacologic effects of these compounds were shown on smooth muscle contraction, cell secretions, and platelet aggregation, which fostered the concept that prostaglandins functioned as local mediators of many biologic systems.

The recognition by Schwarz that the formation of gastroduodenal ulcers is caused by the erosive properties of endogenous gastric acid (Schwarz *dictum: "no acid-no ulcer"*) and that the inhibition of acid secretion enhances ulcer healing, altered the management of this disease from surgery as the mainstay to pharmacologically oriented strategies. Following the discovery of cytoprotective activity of prostaglandins (PGs), stable PG analogs were developed, with the notion that they could play an important role in the pharmacologic treatment of peptic lesions by effectively inhibiting gastric acid secretion in humans. These analogs were found to be effective in accelerating healing ulcer rate not only with associated NSAID therapy, in the presence of an endogenous prostaglandin deficiency, but also in NSAID-independent peptic injury. It was demonstrated that misoprostol (a PGE1 stable analog) significantly decreased the frequency of gastroduodenal ulcers in long-term NSAID users; however, this effect occurred principally as a result of gastric acid inhibition rather than by a cytoprotective mechanism, indicating that cytoprotection plays a lesser role in healing chronic peptic ulcers. Prostaglandins inhibit H^+ ion generation by binding to their EP3 G-protein linked receptor on the parietal cell (see Chapter 2, Figure 2.2), which appears to inhibit adenylate cyclase and thereby decrease intracellular cAMP generation when activated.

Physicochemical properties

Misoprostol, racemic methyl (11a, 13E)-11,16-dihydroxy-16-methyl-9-oxoprost-13-en-1-oate C22H38O5 is a water-insoluble, synthetic prostaglandin E1 (PGE1) analog. The commercially available product is a double racemate of two diastereoisomers containing four stereoisomers prepared in a matrix of hydroxyl propyl methyl cellulose.

Formulations and recommended dosages

Misoprostol tablets (Table 4.1) are commercially available under brand names Cytotec® (100 and 200 µg) and Arthrotec® (enteric-coated core that contains either 50 or 75 mg of diclofenac sodium and an outer layer containing 200 µg misoprostol; originally G.D. Searle, Skokie, IL, and now Pfizer, New York, NY). For patients who need protection from NSAID-induced gastroduodenal mucosal injury, the usual adult dosage

Table 4.1 Data summary of prostaglandins and other mucosal protecting agents

Active	Brand names	Indications	Dosing regimens	Adverse effects
Misoprostol	Arthrotec® Cytotec®	Gastroduodenal ulcer prevention in NSAID chronic users.	200 µg 3–4 times per day with food.	Diarrhea Nausea Abdominal pain Risk of aborption
Sucralfate	Antepsin® Netunal® Indane® Sucralmax® Urbal® Others......	Duodenal ulcer recurrence prevention. Stress ulcer-related bleeding prevention in mechanical ventilated patients. Treatment of heartburn and gastroesophageal reflux in pregnancy.	1gr 4-6 times per day. 8 g maximum dose.	Constipation Nausea Vomiting Diarrhea
Rebamipide	Bamedin® Gaspamin® Mucogen® Mucopid® Others.....	Treatment of NSAID/Hp positive induced gastroduoenal ulcers. Prevention of small bowel NSAID-related injury.	100 mg 3 times per day.	Nausea Vomiting Abdominal pain Upset stomach Myalgia Increased risk of thrombosis

is 200 µg 3–4 times per day, taken with food. For treatment of duodenal ulcer, 4–8 weeks of therapy with 200 µg 4 times per day is recommended. The recommended dosage of Arthrotec is one tablet 2–4 times per day. With all these regimens, the possibility of abdominal cramps and diarrhea, as well as the risk of spontaneous abortion in pregnant women, should be considered. Although not recommended by the manufacturer, to induce abortion, misoprostol is given with other drugs, for example, misoprostol 400–600 µg after RU-496 600 mg once or in two equal divided doses.

Mechanism of action

The antisecretory properties of misoprostol are produced by only one of the diastereoisomeric pairs. Of the two enantiomers making up that diastereoisomeric pair, the 11R, 16S isomer accounts for most, if not all, of the gastric acid antisecretory activity. The presence or lack of stereospecificity of other pharmacologic activities of misoprostol has not been reported. It is reasonable to expect that some effects, such as those derived from misoprostol competing with PGE1 at its binding site, will show significant stereospecificity.

In addition to its antisecretory properties, misoprostol induces marked edema of the mucosa and submucosa. This mucosal edema and increased mucus layer may represent integral components of the drug's cytoprotective mechanisms of action. Edema may dilute the concentration of the gastric secretions and increase the distance that damaging molecules, such as NSAIDs, must penetrate before reaching susceptible cells. Misoprostol, as most commonly administered in the clinical setting, has four dominant effects: gastroduodenal cytoprotection, its approved therapeutic indication, and three side effects, namely, diarrhea, abdominal pain, and uterine contractions. For the optimal delivery of drugs that affect the gastrointestinal tract, it is important to determine whether pharmacologic benefits and toxicity are elicited topically on physical contact or systemically to the site of action after absorption. Convincing animal data indicate that misoprostol's cytoprotective effect occurs principally by topical contact.

Prostaglandins are potent mediators generated in various organs by the enzymatic action of cyclooxygenase on arachidonic acid, and misoprostol, as a prostaglandin analog, might have agonist, antagonist, or both activities relative to endogenous prostaglandins. Misoprostolic acid is an EP2-EP3-selective agonist in intestinal mucosa, preventing the release of a variety of tissue damaging cytokines and inflammatory mediators and by helping to maintain normal homeostasis.

Prostaglandins may exert protective gastrointestinal tract effects by inhibiting the release of platelet-activating factor, tumor necrosis factor (TNF), and histamine from mast cells. It is also likely that misoprostol acts as an inhibitor of leukocyte adherence and/or directly modulates the expression of specific adhesion molecules throughout the body in various disease states. Some of the drug's effects may be due to downregulation of various cytokines. In the presence of lipopolysaccharide (LPS) and human peripheral blood monocytes, 10^{-6} M misoprostol significantly depressed LPS stimulation of interleukin-1, thromboxane B2, and TNF, while further stimulating the production of 6-keto-prostacyclin. A novel delivery system consists of misoprostol molecules attached to a polybutadiene polymer backbone by hydrolyzable covalent bonds. The formulation was designed to release the drug at a controlled rate, but only in an acidic environment. This formulation allowed the release of potentially active misoprostol from the polymer backbone only in the region of the stomach. In addition, whereas the immediate release product caused the expected frequency of diarrhea in test animals, the side effect was negligible after the polymer at all dosages tested in humans. These results indicate that the cytoprotective effects may require little or no drug reaching the systemic circulation and that diarrhea can be eliminated by the combination of very low systemic availability and no release of misoprostol in the intestinal lumen.

Drug interactions

Many studies have evaluated potential interactions between misoprostol and various NSAIDs (aspirin, diclofenac, ibuprofen, indomethacin, piroxicam); however, no clinically significant interactions have been reported to date. The single-dose pharmacokinetics of misoprostolic acid 200 µg did not change significantly when given alone or with aspirin 975 mg. Similarly, no significant differences in ibuprofen and diclofenac pharmacokinetics were detected when administered with misoprostol. Potential pharmacokinetic interactions with other classes of drugs also were investigated. Misoprostol does not change the pharmacokinetics of antipyrine, suggesting that it does not induce hepatic enzymes. Simultaneous administration of misoprostol 800 µg did not cause significant changes in steady-state diazepam and nordiazepam plasma levels. Misoprostol 400 µg twice daily did not alter single-dose or steady-state pharmacokinetics of propranolol given 80 mg twice/day for 2 weeks. One case report suggested a possible increased prothrombin time after 8 days of treatment with a combination of misoprostol 150 µg per day and diclofenac 400 mg per day.

Pharmacokinetics

Misoprostol, an ester, is rapidly and completely de-esterified to pharmacologically active carboxylic acid in the stomach after oral administration. Absorption of misoprostolic acid is rapid, with peak plasma concentration in 15–30 minutes. A 200-µg oral dose produces a peak plasma acid metabolite concentration of 309 ng/L. The acid has a plasma half-life of 20–40 minutes. No detectable concentrations of the parent ester can be found in plasma, and only approximately 7% of the dose is systemically bioavailable as the acid after oral administration. Misoprostol acid is 85% bound to serum albumin plasma protein in a concentration-independent fashion. Misoprostol acid is further metabolized by β-oxidation of the side chain, ω oxidation of the β-side chain, and reduction to prostaglandin F analogs. In addition to undergoing extensive pre-systemic metabolism, misoprostolic acid molecules bind to prostaglandin receptors on parietal cells and to receptors on other gastric and intestinal mucosal cells. The binding may account for some of the clearance of an orally administered dose. The pharmacokinetics of misoprostol are linear, at least within the concentration range achieved after doses of 200–400 µg. Misoprostol fits the criteria of a highly variable drug since it exhibits 43% intersubject variability.

Clinical effectiveness

A Cochrane meta-analysis of 33 randomized-controlled clinical trials of misoprostol, H_2-receptor antagonists (H2RAs) and PPIs revealed that all three classes of drugs reduce the incidence of NSAIDs-related gastroduodenal ulcers. A standard dose of misoprostol (200 µg 4 times per day) was tested in the MUCOSA trial for its ability to reduce NSAID-related ulcer complications, and it proved partially effective (~40% reduction). However, side effects were common and effectively reduced the median daily dose in the study to only about 600 µg. As mentioned above, the properties of misoprostol are mediated to some extent systemically, and its effects are not limited exclusively to the stomach.

NSAIDs can precipitate the development of ulcers and ulcer complications even in patients with achlorhydria, suggesting that prostaglandin replacement therapy would be the ideal approach if it could be offered in a way to minimize side effects. As stated above, misoprostol stimulates mucus secretion and mucosal blood flow and produces other beneficial effects that increase mucosal integrity, effects that occur even at lower doses. Despite its beneficial cytoprotective properties, however, misoprostol is clinically effective only at doses high enough to reduce gastric acid secretion. The effectiveness of misoprostol compared with standard and double doses of PPIs has been confirmed in a study of standard dose misoprostol (200 μg 4 times per day) with two doses of lansoprazole (15 and 30 mg daily) and placebo among 537 *H. pylori*-negative chronic NSAID users with a documented history of gastric ulcer. The study showed that misoprostol was superior for the prevention of gastroduodenal ulcer. For example, at 12 weeks, 93% of patients in the misoprostol group, compared with 80–82% of patients in the two groups receiving lansoprazole, were protected from gastric ulcers. The ulcer rates were 15, 43, and 47 per 100 patient years, for misoprostol, lansoprazole 15 mg, and 30 mg, respectively. However, when the poor compliance and potential side effects associated with misoprostol were considered, PPIs and full-dose misoprostol were clinically equivalent.

Another study compared the effects of omeprazole and misoprostol in preventing ulcer recurrence in arthritic individuals continuing NSAID therapy. In this double-blind, placebo-controlled trial, 732 patients in whom ulcers had healed were randomized to receive either placebo, 20 mg of omeprazole once daily, or 200 μg of misoprostol two times per day as maintenance therapy. After six months, duodenal ulcer was detected in 12 and 10% of those treated with placebo and misoprostol, respectively, while only 3% of those treated with omeprazole developed a duodenal ulcer. Gastric ulcer relapse occurred in 32, 10, and 13% of the individuals receiving placebo, misoprostol, and omeprazole, respectively. These studies provide further evidence that PPIs and misoprostol are similar in their abilities to maintain patients in remission during continued NSAID use.

In a trial that compared misoprostol (200 μg 2–3 times per day) to an H2RA, the former was significantly more effective than ranitidine (150 mg/day) in the short-term prevention of naproxen-induced (500 mg twice daily) gastric ulcers, without differences in the rate of side effects. It is currently not possible to prospectively identify those who will experience symptoms from misoprostol, making a clinical trial the only practical method of identifying those in whom it might be the preferred drug. Because misoprostol and antisecretory agents act via different mechanisms, it is possible that the combination of half-dose misoprostol and an H2RA would provide inexpensive, yet effective, preventive therapy for high-risk patients. Although a PPI would, in theory, represent another similarly effective combination, animal studies have demonstrated that the concomitant use of prostaglandin with a PPI would prevent activation of the PPI prodrug (see above, Chapter 2: Proton pump inhibitors). The fact that the majority of patients took misoprostol without problems in the large clinical trials suggests that individual patients, and not physicians, should decide whether it can be used successfully. Nevertheless, while misoprostol would be in theory superior to therapy aimed at reducing acid secretion only, PPIs have been proven superior to both ranitidine and misoprostol (400 μg per day) in preventing NSAID ulcer recurrence and overall symptom control, largely related to their ability to reduce ulcers and improve NSAID associated dyspepsia, thereby affecting overall quality of life. Therefore, misoprostol is generally not considered a first choice treatment, and the International Consensus Guidelines recommend PPIs as the preferred agents for therapy and prevention of NSAID- and aspirin-related gastroduodenal injury. Misoprostol-induced diarrhea and the need of multiple daily doses (typically four) are the main issues impairing compliance with therapy.

Previous efforts have focused primarily on gastroduodenal ulcers; however, recent efforts have been made to reduce NSAID-induced small bowel and colonic mucosal injury, including mucosal injury, ulceration, overt bleeding, obstruction, perforation, protein-loss, and occult blood loss with associated anemia. One study demonstrated the benefit of treatment with misoprostol in a small pilot study in which small intestinal damage was assessed by capsule endoscopy. Misoprostol co-therapy reduced the incidence of small intestinal lesions induced by a 2-week administration of diclofenac sodium in healthy subjects. Another study examined the therapeutic effect of misoprostol against aspirin-induced injury. The subjects in this study were gastric ulcer patients who were taking low-dose, enteric-coated aspirin. They were treated with a PPI for 8 weeks, but all patients had erythema and erosions in the small intestine shown by capsule endoscopy at 8 weeks. When misoprostol was administered in lieu of a PPI for an additional 8 weeks, small intestinal lesions were improved on the follow-up exam.

Toxicity

In addition to enhancing small bowel motility, prostaglandins activate intestinal chloride channels, leading to chloride-rich fluid secretion that increases luminal sodium and water content and stool hydration. These small bowel alterations can result in abdominal pain and diarrhea, two known side effects of misoprostol and other prosataglandins. A previous meta-analysis showed that misoprostol was associated with a small, but statistically significant, 1.6-fold excess risk of dropout due to drug-induced side effects, and an excess risk of dropouts due to nausea (RR 1.26; 95% CI 1.07 to 1.48), diarrhea (RR 2.36; 95% CI 2.01 to 2.77), and abdominal pain (RR 1.36; 95% CI 1.20 to 1.55). In the MUCOSA trial, 732 of 4404 participants on misoprostol experienced diarrhea or abdominal pain, compared to 399 out of 4439 on placebo, for a relative risk of 1.82 associated with misoprostol (p<0.001). Overall, 27% of participants on misoprostol experienced one or more side effects. When analysed by dose, only misoprostol 800 µg daily showed a statistically significant excess risk of dropouts due to diarrhea (RR 2.45; 95% CI 2.09 to 2.88) or abdominal pain (RR 1.38; 95% CI 1.17 to 1.63). Both misoprostol doses were associated with a statistically significant risk of diarrhea. However, the risk of diarrhea with 800 µg per day (RR 3.16; 95%CI 2.33 to 4.29) was significantly higher than that seen with 400 µg per day (RR 1.76 95% CI 1.37 to 2.26).

Pregnancy classes

MIsoprostol: Cytotec: Category X.
Misoprostol: Arthrotec: Category X.
Category X: Both studies in animals and humans have shown obvious risks to the fetus that clearly outweigh any benefit.

Other mucosal protecting agents

Rebamipide

Rebamipide (Table 4.1) was developed in Japan as a gastroprotective drug and was proven to be superior to cetraxate, the former most-prescribed drug of the same category in the 1980s. It is sold under various names, a list of which can be found at http://www.drugs.com/international/rebamipide.html. The basic mechanisms of action of rebamipide were gradually discerned by a substantial amount of research. The drug appears to induce endogenous prostaglandin expression and to function as an oxygen free radical scavenger. In addtion to these mechanisms, rebamipide appears to possess anti-inflammatory properties, indicating that this agent may regulate physiological defensive functions aimed at maintaining tissue integrity. Accordingly, the term "bioregulation" was coined in 1998 to reflect these properties of rebamipide.

It has been shown that rebamipide induces cyclooxygenase-2 (COX-2) in the rat stomach, which may contribute to the generation of cytoprotective prostaglandins. This drug also stimulates prostaglandin EP4 receptor gene expression, resulting in the stimulation of mucus secretion. It also has been demonstrated to exert its cytoprotective effects by activating epidermal growth factor, stimulating hepatocyte growth factor and improving cell kinetics, and reducing apoptosis and inflammation in several experimental models.

There is some clinical evidence that corroborates the cytoprotective effects of rebamipide in ulcer healing in humans. A randomized, controlled, clinical trial was conducted in Japan to assess the efficacy of rebamipide on ulcer healing and ulcer recurrence in 60 *H. pylori*-positive patients with gastric ulcer. The administration of rebamipide with omeprazole for 8 weeks as an initial therapy significantly improved ulcer healing, decreased neutrophil and mononuclear cells infiltration, and decreased the ulcer recurrence rate compared to omeprazole alone. In a randomized, placebo-controlled, clinical trial also conducted in Japan in healthy volunteers, rebamipide significantly inhibited NSAID-induced gastric mucosal damage, assessed by using a modified Lanza score. More recently, rebamipide 100 mg three times per day for 8 weeks was also shown to be effective and well-tolerated in gastric ulcer healing in NSAID-related and *H. pylori*-infected patients. In a randomized, double blind, placebo-controlled trial including 309 *H. pylori*-related gastric ulcer patients, rebamipide significantly promoted gastric ulcer healing following one week of eradication therapy. Some authors also evaluated the effects of rebamipide in mucosal protection of the lower gastrointestinal tract. A prospective, double-blind study using capsule endoscopy to assess rebamipide in healthy subjects reported that subjects who received diclofenac plus placebo had significantly more mucosal injury in the small intestine compared to those who received diclofenac plus rebamipide. No adverse effects related to rebamipide have been reported in clinical studies.

Sucralfate

Sucralfate (Table 4.1), a sulfated disaccharide, is a basic aluminium salt of sulphated sucrose, which was initially sold under the brand name Carafate® in the USA. It is now sold under many different names, either alone or in combination with other agents (See http://www.medindia .net/drug-price/sucralfate-combination.htm). The drug is minimally absorbed after oral administration and is believed to act primarily at the site of an ulcer by protecting it from the effects of pepsin and acid, and by adsorbing bile salts. Sucralfate is particularly well-tolerated and is nearly free from toxicity. Constipation, the most common side effect, occurs in 2% of patients. When exposed to gastric acid, sucralfate becomes a viscous and adhesive substance that binds selectively and durably to lesions in the gastric and duodenal mucosa. The affinity of sucralfate for defective mucosa is explained by the formation of electrostatic bonds between the negatively charged sucralfate polyanions and the positively charged proteins exuding from lesions. The drug thereby produces a "barrier effect," preventing the penetration of acid, pepsin, and bile salts. It also appears to interfere with the binding of pepsin to the lesions, as well as adsorbing pepsin and bile salts. The drug also stimulates bicarbonate and mucus secretion, as well as the endogenous synthesis of prostaglandin E2 and inhibition of thromboxane release. Sucralfate appears to increase epidermal growth factor binding to ulcerated areas and stimulates macrophage activity.

In the 1990s, sucralfate was evaluated for the treatment of long- and short-term treatment of peptic ulcers due to NSAID use and to *H. pylori* infection and demonstrated to be superior to placebo, but less effective than PPIs. Thus, current guidelines do not recommend sucralfate for this indication. Sucralfate also was tested for radiation proctitis, but a meta-analysis concluded that it cannot be recommended for this indication. Sucralfate has also been used for stress ulcer prophylaxis in critically ill patients, but a recent review concluded only moderate quality of evidence support for the use of H2RAs over sucralfate to prevent bleeding, even considering the potential for an increased risk of nosocomial pneumonia. In patients with mechanical ventilation, H2RAswere reported to offer no benefit compared to sucralfate in preventing stress ulcer-related bleeding, but had higher rates of gastric colonization and ventilator-associated pneumonia. Although little evidence exists, sucralfate has been used as the initial drug in the treatment of heartburn and gastroesophageal reflux in pregnancy after changes in lifestyle are initiated.

Pregnancy classes: Sucralfate: Category B; either animal-reproduction studies have not demonstrated a fetal risk, but there are no controlled studies in pregnant women or animal-reproduction studies have shown an adverse effect (other than a decrease in fertility) that was not confirmed in controlled studies in women in the first trimester (and there is no evidence of a risk in later trimesters).

Recommended reading

Bergstrom S, Danielsson H, Samuelsson B (1964) The enzymatic formation of prostaglandin E2 from arachidonic acid. *Biochem Biophys Acta* **90**: 207–10.

Fujimori S, Seo T, Gudis K, *et al.* (2009) Prevention of nonsteroidal anti-inflammatory drug-induced small-intestinal injury by prostaglandin: a pilot randomized controlled trial evaluated by capsule endoscopy. *Gastrointest Endosc* **69**: 1339–46.

Graham DY, White RH, Moreland LW *et al.* (1993) Duodenal and gastric ulcer prevention with misoprostol in arthritis patients taking NSAID. Misoprostol study group. *Ann Intern Med* **19**: 257–62.

Graham DY, Agrawal NM, Campbell DR, *et al.* (2002) Ulcer prevention in long-term users of nonsteroidal anti-inflammatory drugs: results of a double-blind, randomized, multicenter, active- and placebo-controlled study of misoprostol vs. lansoprazole. *Arch Intern Med* **162**: 169–75.

Hawkey CJ, Karrasch JA, Szczepañski L, Walker DG, Barkun A, Swannell AJ, Yeomans ND (1998) Omeprazole compared with misoprostol for ulcers associated with nonsteroidal antiinflammatory drugs. Omeprazole versus misoprostol for NSAID-induced ulcer management (OMNIUM) study group. *N Engl J Med* **338**: 727–34.
Interesting paper reporting the results of the OMNIUM Study that compared misoprostol and the PPI omeprazole in the treatment and prevention of NSAID-related ulcers.

Huang J, Cao Y, Liao C, Wu L, Gao F (2010) Effect of histamine-2-receptor antagonists versus sucralfate on stress ulcer prophylaxis in mechanically ventilated patients: a meta-analysis of 10 randomized controlled trials. *Crit Care* **14**(5): R194.

Janssen M, Dijkmans BA, Vandenbroucke JP, Biemond I, Lamers CB (1994) Achlorhydria does not protect against benign upper gastrointestinal ulcers during NSAID use. *Dig Dis Sci* **39**: 362–5.

Karim A (1993) Pharmacokinetics of diclofenac and misoprostol when administered alone or as a combination product. *Drugs* **45**(suppl 1): 7–13.

Kleine A, Kluge S, Peskar BM (1993) Stimulation of prostaglandin biosynthesis mediates gastroprotective effect of rebamipide in rats. *Dig Dis Sci* **38**: 1441–9.

Konturek SJ, Kwiecien N, Swierczek J, Oleksy J, Sito E, Robert A (1976) A comparison of methylayed prostaglandin E analogues given orally in the inhibition of gastric responses to pentagastrin and peptone meal in man. *Gastroenterology* **70**: 683–7.

Kurzrok R, Lieb CC (1930) Biochemical studies of human semen-II. The action of semen on the human uterus. *Proc Soc Exp Biol Med* **28**: 268–72.

McCarthy DM (1991) Sucralfate. *N Engl J Med* **325**: 1017–25.
Critical review on the proven value of sucralfate in the treatment of gastroduodenal ulcer and other gastrointestinal disorders. The manuscript includes a detailed evaluation of the various proposed mechanisms of action for sucralfate.

Niwa Y, Nakamura M, Ohmiya N, et al. (2008) Efficacy of rebamipide for diclofenac-induced small-intestinal mucosal injuries in healthy subjects: a prospective, randomized, double-blinded, placebo-controlled, cross-over study. *J Gastroenterol* **43**: 270–6.

Poynard T, Pignon JP (1989) *Acute Treatment of Duodenal Ulcer Analysis of 293 Randomized Clinical Trial.* Paris: John Libbey Eurotext, p. 7.

Rainsford KD, James C, Hunt RH, et al. (1992) Effects of misoprostol on the pharmacokinetics of indomethacin in human volunteers. *Clin Pharmacol Ther* **51**: 415–21.

Robert A, Nezamis JE, Lancaster C, Hanchar AJ (1979) Cytoprotection by prostaglandins in rats. Prevention of gastric necrosis produced by alcohol, HCl, NaOH, hypertonic NaCl and thermal injury. *Gastroenterology* **77**: 433–40.
Important scientific paper showing that prostaglandins possessed cytoprotective properties as evident by their capacity to prevent gastric injury due not only to acid, but to many other noxious agents.

Rostom A, Dube C, Wells G, et al. (2002) Prevention of NSAID-induced gastroduodenal ulcers. *Cochrane Database Syst Rev* **4**: CD002296.

Schaff EA, Eisinger SH, Stadalius LS, Franks P, Gore BZ, Poppema S (1999) Low-dose mifepristone 200 mg and vaginal misoprostol for abortion. *Contraception* **59**: 1–6.

Schoenhard G, Oppermann J, Kohn FE (1985) Metabolism and pharmacokinetic studies of misoprostol. *Dig Dis Sci* **30**(11 suppl): 126S–8.

Silverstein FE, Graham DY, Senior JR, et al. (1995) Misoprostol reduces serious gastrointestinal complications in patients with rheumatoid arthritis receiving nonsteroidal anti-inflammatory drugs. A randomized, double-blind, placebo-controlled trial. *Ann Intern Med* **123**: 241–9.

Important paper that reported the results of the MUCOSA Trial, the first study to evaluate the effects of any agent (in this case, misoprostol) in preventing ulcer bleeding and other complications associated with the use of NSAIDs. Previous studies had focused on endoscopic ulcers rather then clinically relevant outcomes.

Sun WH, Tsuji S, Tsujii M, Gunawan ES, Kawai N, Kimura A, Kakiuchi Y, Yasumaru M, Iijima H, Okuda Y, Sasaki Y, Hori M, Kawano S (2000) Induction of cyclooxygenase-2 in rat gastric mucosa by rebamipide, a mucoprotective agent. *J Pharmacol Exp Ther* **295**: 447–52.

Takemoto T, Namiki M, Yachi A, *et al.* (1989) Effect of rebamipide (OPC-12759) on gastric ulcer healing multicenter, double-blind, cetraxate controlled clinical study. *Rinsho Seijin-byo* **19**: 1265–91.

Tarnawski A, Arakawa T, Kobayashi K (1998) Rebamipide treatment activates epidermal growth factor and its receptor expression in normal and ulcerated gastric mucosa in rats: one mechanism for its ulcer healing action? *Dig Dis Sci* **43**(Suppl): 90S–98S.

Terano A, Arakawa T, Sugiyama T, Suzuki H, Joh T, Yoshikawa T, Higuchi K, Haruma K, Murakami K, Kobayashi K (2007) Rebamipide Clinical Study Group Rebamipide, a gastro-protective and anti-inflammatory drug, promotes gastric ulcer healing following eradication therapy for Helicobacter pylori in a Japanese population: a randomized, double-blind, placebo-controlled trial. *J Gastroenterol Aug.*; **42**(8): 690–3.

Vane JR (1971) Inhibition of prostaglandin synthesis as a mechanism of action for aspirin-like drugs. *Nat New Biol* **231**: 232–5.

Walt RP (1992) Misoprostol for the treatment of peptic ulcer and antiinflammatory-drug-induced gastroduodenal ulceration. *N Engl J Med* **327**: 1575–80.

An excellent review on the use of mispoprostol for treating and preventing gastroduodenal ulcers due to NSAIDs. The paper also discusses the mechanism of action of prostaglandins, indicating that despite their cytoprotective properties, these agents are effective only in doses sufficient to inhibit gastric acid secretion.

Watanabe T, Sugimori S, Kameda N, *et al.* Small bowel injury by low-dose enteric-coated aspirin and treatment with misoprostol: a pilot study. *Clin Gastroenterol Hepatol* **6**: 1279–82.

Wilcox CM, Allison J, Benzuly K, Borum M, Cryer B, Grosser T, Hunt R, Ladabaum U, Lanas A, Paulus H, Regueiro C, Sandler RS, Simon L (2006) American Gastroenterological Association, Consensus development conference on the use of nonsteroidal anti-inflammatory agents, including cyclooxygenase-2 enzyme inhibitors and aspirin. *Clin Gastroenterol Hepatol* **4**: 1082–9.

Yoshikawa T, Arakawa T (1998) *Bioregulation and its Disorders in the Gastrointestinal Tract.* Tokyo: Blackwell Science.

SMALL AND LARGE INTESTINE

PART II

5-HT modulators and other antidiarrheal agents and cathartics

Albena Halpert[1] and Douglas Drossman[2]
[1]Boston University School of Medicine, Boston, MA, USA
[2]Drossman Center for the Education and Practice of Biopsychosocial Care,
Chapel Hill, NC, USA

Introduction

Serotonin (5-hydroxytryptamine or 5-HT) is an important neurotransmitter involved in multiple functions both in the central nervous system and the periphery. Most of the body 5-HT is synthesized in the gastrointestinal (GI) tract, where 5-HT modulates various aspects of intestinal physiology. The wide-ranging effects of serotonin can be explained by the presence of multiple subtypes of 5-HT receptors located on various types of cells (smooth muscle, enteric neurons, enterocytes, and immune cells). Agonist or antagonists of 5-HT receptors are used for the treatment of a range GI disorders (e.g., irritable bowel syndrome, chronic diarrhea, constipation and functional dyspepsia). In addition to 5-HT serotonin agents, there are several other classes of medications used for the treatment of chronic diarrhea and constipation. This chapter will provide information on the clinical use of 5-HT modulators in GI disorders and other anti diarrheal agents and cathartics.

5-HT modulators used in the management of GI disorders

Biology and pharmacology

Serotonin plays a crucial role in the regulation of multiple intestinal functions, including motility, secretion, visceral sensitivity, immune/inflammatory responses, and regulation of the autonomic nervous system. The majority (95%) of the body's serotonin is found in the intestine, with the remainder (5%) residing in CNS neurons and platelets. Within the bowel, serotonin is synthesized from its precursor, amino acid, L–tryptophan,

Pocket Guide to Gastrointestinal Drugs, Edited by M. Michael Wolfe and Robert C. Lowe. © 2014
John Wiley & Sons, Ltd. Published 2014 by John Wiley & Sons, Ltd.

in the enterochromaffin (EC) cell and by serotonergic neurons of the myenteric plexus. Serotonin exerts its effects via neurocrine, paracrine, and endocrine pathways. It acts as a paracrine messenger of the EC cells, which are sensory transducers. Serotonin activates intrinsic and extrinsic primary afferent neurons to initiate peristaltic and secretory reflexes and to transmit information to the central nervous system, respectively. 5-HT inactivation is accomplished by a serotonin reuptake transporter (SERT), which mediates uptake back into the enterocytes or neurons. Serotonin is then metabolized into 5-Hydroxyindole Acetic Acid (5-HIAA).

Serotonin receptors are classified into seven main receptor subtypes, 5-HT1–7, which are present in the gut, Depending on the receptor subtype and its localization, 5-HT evokes different and sometimes opposite responses, explaining its diverse effects on GI function – motility, secretion, absorption and sensation. Clinically, 5-HT$_3$ antagonists alleviate the nausea and vomiting associated with cancer chemotherapy and the abdominal discomfort in irritable bowel syndrome and tend to be constipating. In contrast, 5-HT$_4$ agonists, such as tegaserod, are effective in the treatment of irritable bowel syndrome with constipation and chronic constipation.

The presence of many serotonin receptor subtypes enables selective drugs to be designed to therapeutically modulate gastrointestinal functions. Therapeutic interventions aiming at modulating intestinal 5-HT signaling are mainly focused on the following areas: (1) the development of receptor agonists/antagonists, characterized by high affinity and selectivity for serotonergic receptors in the intestine, to avoid adverse effects in the brain, (2) the use of agents to increase serotonin bioavailability by selectively inhibiting its reuptake, and (3) the use of agents that reduce 5-HT production and release.

Currently available 5-HT agonists and antagonists used in the treatment of GI disorders are presented in Table 5.1. Only a few agents have been specifically approved for GI indications, some are in development stages, and others are used off label. International brand names are listed bellow. The agents approved for specific GI indications will be further discussed in more detail.

5-HT agents approved in the US for specific GI indications

Alosetron

In the United States, Alosetron has been approved for the treatment of women with severe diarrhea-predominant irritable bowel syndrome who failed to respond to conventional treatment. The efficacy and safety of Alosetron at a dose of 1 mg twice daily for 12 weeks vs. placebo was determined based on a total of 1273 nonconstipated women with IBS. The

Table 5.1 5-HT agonists and antagonists

Class	Compound	GI effects	Clinical application	Brand names and dose	Major side effects	Major contra-indications pregnancy category
5-HT₁ agonists	**Buspirone**	Improves proximal gastric accommodation Slows gastric emptying	Functional dyspepsia (FD), specifically post-prandial distress (PDS) **(off label)**	US : Buspar® 15 mg/day (7.5 mg bid); maximum 60 mg/day.	Dizziness drowsiness headache, nervousness	Hypersensitivity to Buspirone; not recommended in: severe renal or hepatic impairment; concurrent use of MAO inhibitors **Pregnancy category B;** Not studied in **children <6 years** of age
	Sumatriptan	Enhances gastric accommodation, motility, and visceral sensitivity	Not established			
	R-137696	Improves proximal gastric accommodation; stimulates interdigestive phase 3	Not established			

(continued)

Table 5.1 (*Continued*)

Class	Compound	GI effects	Clinical application	Brand names and dose	Major side effects	Major contra-indications pregnancy category
5-HT$_3$ agonists	MKC-733	Stimulation of interdigestive phase 3; increases small bowel transit; slows emptying of liquids	Not established			
5-HT$_3$ antagonists	Alosetron	Inhibits responses to intestinal distention; decreases colonic tone; delays colonic transit; affects the regulation of visceral pain, colonic transit, and GI secretions	Women with severe IBS-D who failed to respond to conventional therapy	US: Lotronex® International : not available Initial: 0.5 mg bid for 4 weeks, if tolerated, but if response is inadequate, may be increased after 4 weeks to 1 mg bid. If response is inadequate after 4 weeks of 1 mg bid, discontinue treatment.	Constipation, which is dose-related (9%–29%); fatigue, headache, bdominal pain, nausea, ischemic colitis *US boxed warning: Acute ischemic colitis has been reported during treatment.*	Constipation. History of ischemic colitis, intestinal obstruction, stricture, toxic megacolon, gastrointestinal perforation, adhesions, diverticulitis, Crohn's disease, ulcerative colitis, severe hepatic impairment, impaired intestinal circulation, thrombophlebitis, or hypercoagulable

		Should only be prescribed by physicians enrolled in the Prometheus Prescribing Program for Lotronex®. Patients must read and sign a "patient-physician" agreement before receiving the initial prescription	*Discontinue immediately in patients who develop constipation*	state, severe hepatic impairment, patients unable to understand or comply with "Patient-Physician" agreement, concomitant administration with fluvoxamine *Pregnancy category B;* Not studied in *children*
Ondansetron	Blocks 5HT$_3$, peripherally on vagal nerve terminals and centrally in the chemoreceptor trigger zone; inhibits nausea; slows small bowel transit; improves	Nausea and vomiting associated with chemotherapy, radiotherapy, and postoperative; hyperemesis gravidarum (severe or refractory) – **off label**	US: Zofran®; Zofran® ODT; Zuplenz® IV: 0.15-16 mg/kg/dose prior to chemotherapy Oral 8-24 mg prior and during chemotherapy Children: weight based dosing	Anxiety, dizziness, constipation, diarrhea, urinary retention, liver enzyme elevation, injection site reaction, paresthesia, hypoxia Rare: arrhythmias,	Hypersensitivity to ondansetron, other 5-HT$_3$ receptor antagonists, concurrent use of apomorphine Special warning : QT Prolongation

(continued)

Table 5.1 (*Continued*)

Class	Compound	GI effects	Clinical application	Brand names and dose	Major side effects	Major contra-indications pregnancy category
5-HT$_3$ antagonists (*continued*)	**Ondansetron** (*continued*)	Increases stool consistency and tends to delay colonic transit			QT interval prolongation; torsades de pointes; atrial fibrillation, AV block, transient blindness	**Pregnancy category B; Children:** weight based dosing
	Granisetron	Enteric interneurons and secreto-motor neurons; inhibits opiate-induced nausea Decreases intestinal secretion reduces rectal sensitivity and postprandial motility	Prevention of chemotherapy-associated and postoperative nausea and vomiting	U.S.Granisol™, Sancuso® i.v 10 mcg/kg/dose (max 1 mg/dose) Oral: 2 mg daily or 1 mg bid **Children:** age-based dosing	Headache, constipation, weakness, QT prolongation, anxiety, liver enzyme elevation	Hypersensitivity to granisetron, other 5-HT$_3$ antagonists; Warning dose-dependent increases in ECG intervals (e.g. PR, QRS duration, QT/QT$_c$ **Pregnancy category B; Children:** age based dosing
	Palonosetron	Antagonizes the 5-HT$_3$ receptors located on vagal afferents, which initiate the vomiting reflex triggered by chemotherapy agents	Prevention of chemotherapy-associated and postoperative nausea and vomiting;	U.S. Aloxi® 0.25 mg IV 30 minutes before the start of chemotherapy.	QT prolongation, hypotension, Arrhythmias, Headache, hyperkalemia, Constipation, elevated liver enzymes	Hypersensitivity to palonosetron; Warning: ECG effects **Pregnancy category B; Children:** weight based dosing

Cilansetron	Inhibits colonic response to feeding; slows colonic transit	IBS-D	Not FDA approved	Severe constipation and ischemic colitis
Ramosetron	Blocks 5-HT$_3$ receptors present in the afferent vagal nerve endings in the GI mucosa.	IBS-D; Prevention of chemotherapy-associated nausea and vomiting;	Not available in USA Nausea 100 mcg po once daily. 0.3 mg iv daily IBS-D in men 5 mcg once daily, may adjust dose according to symptoms. Max: 10 mcg/day	Headache, diarrhea, constipation, rash, itching, redness, heat, hot flashes, hiccup, hepatic dysfunction, increased BUN	Hypersensitivity to Ramosetron Safety in **pregnancy** and **children** has not been evaluated
5-HT$_4$ antagonists				
Prucalopride	Enhances acetylcholine release from colonic motor neurons; increases colonic transit; no effect on gastric or small bowel transit	Chronic idiopathic constipation in adult females with inadequate response to laxatives; opioid-induced constipation in chronic pain (non cancer) patients-off label	Not available in USA 2 mg p.o daily.	Headache (22%), nausea, vomiting, diarrhea; Warning ECG effects and ischemic colitis	Hypersensitivity to prucalopride **Pregnancy category:** unknown. Reproductive animal studies did not demonstrate adverse effects. Contraception recommended; Use not recommended in **children** <18 years of age.

(continued)

Table 5.1 (Continued)

Class	Compound	GI effects	Clinical application	Brand names and dose	Major side effects	Major contra-indications pregnancy category
5-HT₄ antagonists (*continued*)	**Tegaserod**	Stimulation of the peristaltic reflex and intestinal secretion, and moderation of visceral sensitivity. accelerates gastric emptying and small bowel transit	Treatment of (IBS-C) and chronic idiopathic constipation (CIC) in women (<55 years of age) in whom no alternative therapy exists	Zelnorm® 6 mg bid 30 min before meals *Available in USA. under an emergency investigational new drug (IND) process*	Headache (15%) Abdominal pain (12%)	Hypersensitivity to tegaserod severe renal impairment; moderate or severe hepatic impairment; history of bowel obstruction, symptomatic gallbladder disease, suspected sphincter of Oddi dysfunction, or abdominal adhesions, patients with diarrhea. Exclusion criteria under the emergency-IND process: unstable angina, history of MI or stroke, hypertension, hyperlipidemia, diabetes, age ≥55 years, smoking, obesity, depression, anxiety, or suicidal ideation. **Pregnancy category B;** Safety and efficacy have not been established in males and **children**

| Mixed 5-HT$_4$ agonists/ 5-HT$_3$ antagonists | Cisapride | Enhances the release of acetylcholine from myenteric plexus; may increase GI motility and heart rate; increases lower esophageal sphincter pressure and lower esophageal peristalsis; accelerates gastric emptying of both liquids and solids | Nocturnal symptoms of GERD; gastroparesis, chronic constipation; dyspepsia | US Propulsid® available only under compassionate – release program/ limited-access protocol) 5–10 mg 4 times/ day before meals, maximum 20 mg/ dose; Children: 0.15–0.3 mg/ kg/dose 3–4 times/ day; maximum: 10 mg/dose | Headache (> 10%), Diarrhea (>10 %), tachycardia, fatigue, anxiety, constipation | Hypersensitivity to cisapride; GI hemorrhage; mechanical obstruction; GI perforation; serious cardiac arrhythmias, including ventricular tachycardia, ventricular fibrillation, torsade de pointes, and QT prolongation; concomitant use of erythromycin, clarithromycin, troleandomycin, nefazodone, fluconazole, itraconazole, miconazole, oral ketoconazole, indinavir, ritonavir, amprenavir, atazanavir **Pregnancy category C; Children:** weight based dosing |
| | Renzapride | Increases small bowel and colonic transit | IBS M IBS-C Chronic idiopathic constipation | Phase III | | |

(continued)

Table 5.1 (*Continued*)

Class	Compound	GI effects	Clinical application	Brand names and dose	Major side effects	Major contra-indications pregnancy category
Mixed 5-HT₄ agonists/ 5-HT₃ antagonists (*continued*)	**Mosapride**	Increases gastric emptying	IBS-M IBS-C Chronic idiopathic constipation	Not available in USA International 5 mg po tid	Diarrhea abdominal pain, dizziness, constipation, headache, sleeplessness, nausea and vomiting	Hypersensitivity to Mosapride, history of liver or kidney impairment, **Pregnancy category:** unknown use during pregnancy; not recommended; Use in **children** not recommended

IBS-D Irritable bowel syndrome diarrhea predominant
IBS-C Irritable bowel syndrome constipation predominant
IBS-M Irritable bowel syndrome mixed type
GERD gastroesophageal reflux disease; FDA US Food and Drug Administration

International brand names for **Buspirone**
Actium, Ansial, Ansitec, Anxiolan, Anxiron, Anxut, Bespar, Buporin, Busiral, Busp, Buspar, Busparium, Buspin, Buspon, Dalpas, Dergelasen; Kallmiren, Normaton, Pasrin, Paxon, Relac, Sepirone, Sorbon, Spamilan, Spitomin, Suxin, Travin, Xiety

International brand names for Ondansetron

Apo-Ondansetron®, CO Ondansetron, Dom-Ondansetron, JAMP-Ondansetron, Mint-Ondansetron, Mylan-Ondansetron, Ondansetron Injection USP, Ondansetron-Odan, Ondansetron-Omega, PHL-Ondansetron; PMS-Ondansetron, RAN™-Ondansetron, ratio-Ondansetron, Sandoz-Ondansetron, Teva-Ondansetron, Zofran®, Zofran® ODT, ZYM-Ondansetron, Zofran, Zofran Zydis Avessa

Cedantron, Cetron, Danac, Dantron, Danzetron, Emeset, Emetron, Emistop, Emodan, Frazon, Glotron, Invomit, Izofran, Lartron, Modifical, Narfoz; Nausedron, Ondak, Ondant Ondavell, Ondaz, Onetic, Onset-8, Onsetron, Onsia, Onzod, Osetron, Setronax, Vomceran, Vometron, Vomiof, Vomiz;

Zetron, Zofron, Zophren

International brand names for Granisetron

Granisetron Hydrochloride Injection; Kytril, Gramet, Granicip, Granon, Grantron, Helminar, Kanitron, Kevatril, Kyotil; Neosetron, Nisetron, Sancuso, Patch, Setron, Sulingqiong

International brand names for Palonosetron

Aloxi, Lowvo, Onicit, Paloxi, Palzen, Zhirvo

International brand names for Ramosetron

Ai Ke An, Lei Mai Xin, Nasea, Nasea OD, Setoral, Shan Cheng, Irribow

International brand names for Prucalopride

Resotran, Resolor, Resotrans

International brand names for Tegaserod

Colonaid, Coloserod, Gasprid, Prozerada, Tegibs, Zelmac, Zelnorm

International brand names for Cisapride

Acenalin, Acpulsif, Alimix, Alimix Forte, Alipride, Cipasid, Cisamod, Cisaride, Cisawal, Coordinax, Cyprid; Digenol, Disflux; Enteropride, Esorid; Gasprid, Gastromet; Kinestase; Lornakin; Pepta, Prepulsid, Presistin, Prider, Pridesia, Profercol, Pulsar; Refluxin, Risamol; Stimulit; Tadasil; Unamol; Viprasen, Vomipride

International brand names for Mosapride

Kinetix Tab, Mic Tab, Mopride Tab, Mosadec 5 Tab, Mosafe Film-Coated Tab, Mosagen Tab, Mosakind Tab, Mosap Tab, Mosapid Tab, Mosiba Tab, Mosid-Mps Tab, Mosid-Mt Mel-Tab, Mosid-Od Tab, Moten Instab Tab, Moza Mps Tab, Moza Plus Cap, Moza Sr-Tab, Moza Tab, Mozasef Tab, Mozatone Tab, Mozax Mel-Tab, Mozax-Mps Tab, M-Pride Tab, Musapro Tab, Muzic Tab, Normagut Tab, Remo Tab. Biotonus, Gastride, Mosad OD/Mosad MT, Mosart, Reflucil, Safepride, Dosier, Galopran, Gasmotin, Intesul, Lostapride, Mosar, Mosid, Motigest, Moxar, Moza, Mozax, Vagantyl

primary endpoints of the placebo-controlled trials were adequate relief of pain and discomfort, which was assessed weekly. Secondary endpoints were the percentage of days with urgency and daily assessment of stool frequency and consistency. An additional study compared alosetron (1 mg twice daily) to mebeverine, an antispasmodic approved in Europe for the treatment of IBS. Because of the rare, but serious, side effect of ischemic colitis observed in the clinical trials and early post-marketing surveillance of alosetron, the drug was voluntarily withdrawn from the US marketplace in December 2000. In 2002, it was re-released for monitored use. Physicians must enroll in the Prometheus Prescribing Program for Lotronex® (www. lotronexppl.com or 1-888-423-5227) in order to prescribe this medication.

Tegaserod

Tegaserod is a highly selective partial 5-HT$_4$ agonist. Its action at the receptor site leads to stimulation of the peristaltic reflex and intestinal secretion and moderation of visceral sensitivity. Clinical trials have demonstrated that Tegaserod at a dose of 6 mg bid provides significant improvement in the global assessment of IBS symptoms and in individual symptoms, such as abdominal pain, bloating, and bowel habits, in women with IBS-C when compared with placebo, Due to cardiovascular side effects, in the USA Tegaserod is approved by the FDA for restrictive use, under an emergency investigational new drug (IND) process, only in the emergency treatment of irritable bowel syndrome with constipation (IBS-C) and chronic idiopathic constipation (CIC) in women (<55 years of age) in whom no alternative therapy exists. Emergency situations are defined as immediately life-threatening or requiring hospitalization. Physicians with patients who may qualify can contact the FDA's Division of Drug Information via email (druginfo@fda.hhs.gov). Additional information can be found at http://www.fda.gov/Drugs/DrugSafety/PostmarketDrugSafetyInformationforPatientsandProviders/ucm103223.htm.

Medications increasing serotonin bioavailability

Selective serotonin reuptake inhibitors (SSRIs), indicated for the treatment of depression, increase serotonin bioavailability by selectively inhibiting its reuptake. These agents modulate GI function independent of its antidepressant properties and are used off label for the management of functional GI disorders. Despite clinical evidence for their efficacy in IBS, there is limited and often conflicting research data. Available data involves mostly fluoxetine and citalopram. Fluoxetine was shown to significantly reduce abdominal discomfort and a feeling of bloating, increase frequency of bowel movements, and improve overall well-being. As a serotonin-enhancing agent, diarrhea may occur as a side effect. For patients with severe IBS, both psychotherapy and paroxetine have been shown to improve health-related quality of life at no additional cost. Another SSRI, Citalopram, was shown to improve the severity of IBS symptoms, including pain in non-depressed IBS patients. Changes in pain were independent of changes in anxiety or depression, suggesting that SSRIs may have peripheral benefits.

Other medications modulating 5-HT

LX1031 and LX1033 are tryptophan hydroxylase (TPH) inhibitors, which reduce 5-HT production and release, thereby acting as a 5-HT antagonist. In a recent study, LX1031 (250 mg or 1000 mg given qid) was shown to improve abdominal pain and diarrhea in nonconstipated patients with IBS. Improvement correlated inversely with 5-HIAA urinary secretion, thus showing proof of concept and the possibility that 5-HIAA levels may be a biomarker for the clinical response of this agent. Currently, LX1033 a more potent TPH inhibitor, is under investigation as well.

Medications used for the treatment of chronic constipation

Constipation is a disorder characterized by unsatisfactory defecation, which is associated with hard, infrequent stools, difficult stool passage, or both, and is broadly divided into primary (chronic idiopathic constipation, CIC) and secondary constipation. Pharmacologic treatments for chronic constipation include several groups of medications with different mechanism/mode of action as outlined bellow. Specific doses and side effects are presented in Table 5.2.

Bulk-forming agents are organic polymers that absorb water and thus increase stool mass and water content, thereby making it bulkier, softer, and easier to pass. These agents are often used as the first-line treatment of mild constipation.

Stool softeners are surface-active agents that facilitate water interacting with the stool in order to soften the stool, make it more slippery, and easier to pass.

Osmotic laxatives are poorly absorbed ions or molecules that create an osmotic gradient within the intestinal lumen, drawing water into the lumen and making stools soft and loose. These agents are usually used for short-term treatment of constipation or for intermittent use in chronic constipation. PEG solution is also used for intestinal purges in preparation for diagnostic procedures (e.g., colonoscopy) or surgery.

Stimulant laxatives increase peristalsis in the large bowel and fluid and electrolyte secretion in the distal small bowel and colon. These agents are usually used for intermittent and short-term treatment of constipation.

Chloride channel activating secretory agents – this group is currently represented by Lubiprostone, a chloride channels activator, leading to chloride-rich intestinal fluid secretion that increases luminal sodium and water content and stool hydration.

Table 5.2 Agents for treatment of chronic constipation*

Class	Usual dose in adults	Side effects	OTC/RX
Bulk forming agents			
Psyllium	3.5 gm up to tid	Bloating/Gas	OTC
Mrhylcellulose	2 gm up to tid		Pregnancy: considered
Polycharbophil	2–4 tab/day		safe for occasional use
Wheat dextrin	1–3 gm po up to tid		with adequate liquids; used in children
Stool softeners/ surfactants			
Docusate sodium	100 mg bid	Abdominal cramping, bloating, diarrhea, nausea, vomiting, perianal irritation. Palpitations	OTC Pregnancy: short term use considered safe; used in children
Docusate calcium	240 mg qd	Abdominal cramping, bloating, diarrhea, nausea, vomiting, perianal irritation. Palpitations	OTC Pregnancy: short- term use considered safe; used in children
Osmotic laxatives			
Polyethylene glycol	17 gm qd	Nausea, bloating, cramping	OTC **Pregnancy category C;** In children (unlabeled use) widely used in US, although FDA approved for treatment of occasional constipation in ages >17

Class	Usual dose in adults	Side effects	OTC/RX
Lactulose	10–20 gm (15 to 30 ml) dq	Abdominal bloating, flatulence	RX **Pregnancy category B;** In children, FDA approved for treatment of portal systemic encephalopathy; for constipation, FDA approved for adults only.
Sorbitol	30 gm qd	Abdominal bloating, flatulence	OTC FDA approved in ages ≥12 years and adults
Glycerin	2 gm (1 supp) per rectum qd	Rectal irritation	OTC children FDA approved in ages ≥2 years
Magnesium sulfate	5-10 gm qd	Caution in renal insufficiency and CHF	OTC children approved for use in indications other than constipation (e.g., seizures)
Magnesium citrate	200 ml (11.5 gm) qd		OTC Children: short-term treatment of constipation
Stimulant laxatives			
Bisacodyl	10–30 mg po 10 mg supp per rectum qd	Gastric or rectal irritation	OTC children: short-term treatment of constipation
Senna	15–30 mg /day	Melanosis coli	OTC children: short-term treatment of constipation
Other			
Mineral oil	15–45/ml/day	Aspiration: lipid pneumonitis avoid in elderly	OTC Not recommended in pregnancy; used in children

(continued)

Table 5.2 *(Continued)*

Class	Usual dose in adults	Side effects	OTC/RX
Chloride channel activators			
Lubiprostone	8 mcg po bid for IBS-C and 24 mcg po bid for CC	Nausea, diarrhea, abdominal pain, chest tightness, dyspnea	RX **Pregnancy category C;** Not evaluated in children
Guanylate cyclase receptor agonist	IBS-C: 290 mcg taken orally once daily on an empty stomach.	Diarrhea, abdominal pain, flatulence and abdominal distension	RX **Pregnancy category C;** US. boxed warning: Use is contraindicated in pediatric patients ≤6 years of age.
Linaclotide	CIC: 145 mcg taken orally once daily on an empty stomach		Avoid use in pediatric patients 6–17 years of age
5-HT4 Agonists			
Tegaserod	Information in Table 1		
Bacteriotherapy			
Probiotics	1 tab/day– multiple preparations/ strains of probiotics available	Occasional abdominal bloating	OTC; Not studied in pregnancy; not regulated by the FDA

*Listing US and international brand names for all fiber supplements, over the counter laxatives and probiotics is beyond the scope of this chapter. Listed below are selected examples:

Brand names for fiber supplements:

Psyllium: Bulk-K [OTC]; Fiberall® [OTC]; Fibro-Lax [OTC]; Fibro-XL [OTC]; Hydrocil® Instant [OTC]; Konsyl-D™ [OTC]; Konsyl® Easy Mix™ [OTC]; Konsyl® Orange [OTC]; Konsyl® Original [OTC]; Konsyl® [OTC]; Metamucil® Plus Calcium [OTC]; Metamucil® Smooth Texture [OTC]; Metamucil® [OTC]; Natural Fiber Therapy Smooth Texture [OTC]; Natural Fiber Therapy [OTC]; Reguloid [OTC]

Methylcellulose: Citrucel® [OTC]; Soluble Fiber Therapy [OTC Bulk (AT); International: Celevac; Cellulone; Citrucel; Cologel; Dacryolarmes; Davilose; Lacril; Lacrisyn; Methylcellulose-Bournonville; Muciplasma; Oftan MC; Tear cell

Polycharbophil: Equalactin®; Fiber-Lax; Fiber-Tabs™; FiberCon®; Fibertab; Konsyl® Fiber Fibercon; Fiberphil; Mitrolan; Sylcon

Wehat Dextrin: Benefiber® Plus Calcium [OTC]; Benefiber® [OTC]

Internaional brand names for Docusate: Coloxyl; Cusate; Dama-Lax; Dioctyl; Docusaat; Docusoft; Docusol; Doslax; Emtix; Irwax; Jamylene; Klyx; Lambanol; Laxadine; Laxol; Molcer; Norgalax; Norgalax Micro-enema; Otowax; Pedia-lax Liquid Stool Softener; Purgeron; Regutol; Soliwax; Soluwax Ear Drops; Tirolaxo; Wasserlax; Waxsol; Yi Ke Long

Brand names for Polyethylene glycol: Dulcolax Balance® [OTC]; MiraLAX® [OTC]

International names for Sorbitol: Agarol; Ardeanutrisol SO; Cystosol; klysma Sorbit; Medevac; Progras; Resulax; Sladial; Sorbilande; Sorbilax; Sorbit Fresenius; Sorbit Leopold; Sorbit Mayrhofer; Sorbitol Aguettant; Sorbitol Baxter; Sorbitol Delalande; Sorbitol-Infusionslosung; Syn M.D.

International brand names for Glycerin: Babylax; Bebegel; Bulboid; Cristal; Czopki Glicerolowe; Czopki Glicerynowe; Farmino; Formula Liquida Limpieza; Gely; Glicerina; Glicerina Cinfa; Glicerina Quimpe; Glicerine; Glicerol Vilardell; Glicerolo; Glicerolo Dynacren; Glicerolo Sofar; Glicerolo supposte; Glicerotens; Glycerin Suppositories; Glycerinzapfchen Sanova; Glycerinzapfchen Sokosi; Glycerol Suppositories BP; Glycerol "Oba"; Glycerotone; Glycilax; Glyzerinzapfchen Rosch; Jabon de glicerina; Jabon Dermic; Kimos; Luxoral; Micronema; Milax; Miniderm; Nene-Lax; Neotomic; Neutrobar; Obifax; Practomil; Q.V. Wash Soap Free Cleansing Liquid; RubieLax; Supo Glicerina Brota; Supo Glicerina Cinfa; Supo Glicerina Cuve; Supo Glicerina Orravan; Supo Glicerina Orto; Supo Glicerina Rovi; Supo Glicerina Torrent; Supo Glicerina Vilardell; Supo Glicerina Viviar; Supo Gliz; Supo Kristal; Supos Glicerina Mandri; Supositorios de Glicerina Fecofar; Supositorios de Glicerina Parke-Davis; Suppositoria Glycerini; Supposte Glicerina Carlo Erba; Supposte Glicerina S.Pellegrino; Supposte Glicerolo AD-BB Sofar Verolax; Vitrosups; Zetalax

Brand and international names for Senna: Black Draught®; Evac-U-Gen®; ex-lax® Maximum Strength; ex-lax®; Fleet® Pedia-Lax™ Quick Dissolve; Fletcher's®; Geri-kot; Little Tummys® Laxative; Perdiem® Overnight Relief; Senexon®; Senna-Lax; SennaGen; Senokot® Agiolax; Bekunis; Bekunis Krauter; Bekunis Senna; Sennalax; Senokot

International names for Magnesium Citrate: Argocytromag; Citramag; Magnesol; Usanimals

International names for Magnesium Sulfate: Cholal modificado; Inj. Magnesii Sulfurici;Kiddi Pharmaton; Magnesii Sulfas; Magnesii Sulfas Siccatus; Magnesium Sulfuricum; Magunesin; Vivioptal Junior

International names for Bisacodyl: Alophen®; Bisac-Evac™; Biscolax™; Correctol® Tablets; Dacodyl™; Doxidan®; Dulcolax®; ex-lax® Ultra; Femilax™; Fleet® Bisacodyl; Fleet® Stimulant Laxative; Veracolate®; Apo-Bisacodyl®; Bisacodyl-Odan; Bisacolax; Carter's Little Pills®; Codulax; Dulcolax®; PMS-Bisacodyl; ratio-Bisacodyl; Silver Bullet Suppository; Soflax; The Magic Bullett; Woman's Laxative

Brand and international names for Lubiprostone: Amitiza; Lubowel

Brand name for Linaclotide: Linzess

Prokinetic agents – These agents act by increasing intestinal motility and thereby accelerating intestinal transit. Tegaserod maleate is a 5-HT$_4$ receptor agonist, which has been discussed above under 5-HT modulators.

Guanylate cyclase agonists – Linaclotide is a guanylate cyclase agonist that stimulates intestinal fluid secretion and transit. Linaclotide has been approved by the FDA for treatment of IBS with constipation.

With the exception of lubiprostone, linaclotide, and lactulose (and previously, tegaserod maleate), drugs for chronic constipation are available without a prescription (i.e., OTC). They are given one to three times daily and typically work within 12 hours to 1 week. Table 5.2 summarizes the most common products available in the US.

Bacteriotherapy – Probiotics suppress the growth of pathogenic bacteria and modulate the immune system and pain perception. However, most studies have been small and with other limitations. In addition, considerable differences exist in composition, doses, and biologic activity among various commercial preparations, so that results with one preparation cannot be applied to all probiotic preparations. Various preparations are now used for diarrhea, constipation, and IBS and are not FDA regulated.

Medications used for the treatment of narcotic-induced constipation

Narcotics are used commonly as analgesics in many conditions, such as during the postoperative period and to relieve pain associated with malignancies. These exogenous opioids decrease peristalsis and the secretion of fluid and electrolytes into the intestinal lumen, thereby causing constipation, which can be severe and lead to prolonged hospitalization and morbidity. In addition to laxatives and stool-softening agents, two agents are specifically approved by the FDA for opioid-induced constipation – lubiprostone and methylnaltrexone (Restilor®). As discussed above, the former is a chloride channels activator and is used at a dose of 24 mcg orally twice daily. Methylnaltrexone is a mu-opioid receptor antagonist that does not cross the blood-brain barrier and therefore does not interfere with the analgesic effects of opioids. It is administered by subcutaneous injection at a dose of 8 or 12 mg every other day to a maximum of one dose per 24 hours. With the exception of occasional abdominal pain, nausea, and diarrhea, the drug is fairly well-tolerated and has been assigned to pregnancy class B.

Antidiarrheal agents

Several classes of agents are used for symptomatic relive of acute or chronic diarrhea (Table 5.3). Disease-specific treatment, if an underlying diagnosis is made, may be indicated (e.g., antibiotics for infectious

Table 5.3 Medications used for symptomatic treatment of diarrhea

Agent / brand name	Mechanism of action	Clinical use	Dose	Common side effects	Contraindications pregnancy category
Loperamide **OTC** US Imodium, K-Pek II, NeoDiaral, Diaraid	Synthetic opioid. Acts directly on circular and longitudinal intestinal muscles, through the opioid receptor, to inhibit peristalsis and prolong transit time; reduces fecal volume, increases viscosity, and diminishes fluid and electrolyte loss; demonstrates antisecretory activity. Increases tone on the anal sphincter. No CNS effects in therapeutic doses	Control and symptomatic relief of chronic diarrhea associated with inflammatory bowel disease and of acute nonspecific diarrhea; to reduce volume of ileostomy discharge OTC labeling: Control of symptoms of diarrhea, including Traveler's diarrhea Off label: Cancer treatment-induced diarrhea (e.g., irinotecan- induced); chronic diarrhea caused by bowel resection	Adults Max 16 mg /day Children weight-based dosing	Dizziness, fatigue, abdominal pain, constipation nausea, dry mouth	Hypersensitivity, bloody diarrhea, high fever, infectious diarrhea, pseudomembranous colitis **Pregnancy category C**

(continued)

Table 5.3 (*Continued*)

Agent / brand name	Mechanism of action	Clinical use	Dose	Common side effects	Contraindications pregnancy category
Cholestyramine (Rx) US Prevalite, Questran, Questran Light, LoCholest	Forms a nonabsorbable complex with bile acids in the intestine, releasing chloride ions in the process; inhibits enterohepatic reuptake of intestinal bile salts, thereby increasing the fecal loss of bile salt-bound low density lipoprotein cholesterol	Diarrhea associated with excess fecal bile acids **(off label)**	3–4 g 3–4 times / day to a maximum of 16–32 g/day in 2–4 divided doses; Children weight-based dosing	Constipation (20%), heartburn abdominal pain, nausea/vomiting	Hypersensitivity to bile-sequestering resins, complete biliary obstruction. Cautions: renal impairment, concomitant spironolactone use; may interfere with fat absorption and decrease absorption of fat soluble vitamins (A, D, E, K); pre-existing constipation. Take other drugs at least 1 hr before or 4–6 hr after taking cholestyramine to minimize possible interference with absorption **Pregnancy category C**

| Lomotil diphenoxylate US: Lomotil® | Diphenoxylate is an opioid that inhibits excessive GI motility and GI propulsion; commercial preparations contain a subtherapeutic amount of atropine to discourage abuse | Inhibits excessive GI motility and GI propulsion | 5 mg 4 times/day, max 20 mg/day Pediatric weight-based dosing | Confusion, depression, dizziness, drowsiness, flushing, headache, hyperthermia, lethargy, malaise, restlessness, sedation, nausea, pancreatitis, paralytic ileus, toxic megacolon, vomiting, xerostomia, urinary retention | Hypersensitivity to diphenoxylate, atropine, or any component of the formulation; obstructive jaundice Diarrhea associated with pseudomembranous enterocolitis or enterotoxin-producing bacteria; not for use in children <2 years of age **Pregnancy category C** |

International brand names for **Loperamide**
Amerol, Arestal, Beamodium, Betaperamide, Binaldan, Colidium, Colifilm, Coliper, Stop-ratiopharm, Diadium;Diamide, Diaperol, Diarlop, Diarodil, Diatabs, Diatrol, Dissenten, Donafan, Dyspagon,Elcoman, Fortasec, Gastro-Stop, Gastron, Harmonise, Imodium, Imodonil, Imonox, Imosec, Imosen, Imossel, Lenide-T, Lodia, Lomotil, Lopamide, Lopedin, Lopedium, Lopemid, Loper, Loperamid-ratiopharm, Loperamide-Eurogenerics, Loperamide-Generics, Loperamil, Loperhoe, Loperium, Lopermid, Lopermide, Lopicare, Lopmin, Loprex, Loramide, Luobaomai, Motilex, NT-Diorea; Pangetan, Perasian, Permid, Regulane, Rexamide, Reximide, Rhomuz, Safe, Salvacolina, Sanpo, Seldiar, Shilshul, Stopit, Suprasec, Toban, Toban F, Undiarrhea, Vacontil, Velaral; Apo-Loperamide, Diarr-Eze, Dom-Loperamide, Loperacap, Novo-Loperamide, PMS-Loperamide, Rhoxal-loperamide, Rho®-Loperamine, Riva-Loperamide; Sandoz-Loperamide

International brand names for **Cholestyramine**
Choles, Colestiramina, Colestrol, Kolestran, Lipocol-Merz, Quantalan, Quantalan Zuckerfrei, Questran, Questran Light, Questran Loc, Resincolestiramina; Semide, Sequest, Vasosan, Vasosan P-Granulat, Vasosan S-Granulat

International brand names for **Diphenoxylate**
Beamotil, Dhamotil, Diarase, Diarsed, Diastop, Dimotil, Diphenoxylate A, Lofenoxal, Lomotil, Lomotine Reasec

diarrhea or 5-ASA preparations for inflammatory bowel disease). Symptom-directed treatments are contraindicated if diarrhea is accompanied by high fever or blood in the stool or when inhibition of peristalsis is undesirable or dangerous.

Conclusion

In conclusion, most 5-HT modulating agents used in the treatment of GI disorders are used off label or under restricted prescribing programs (at least in the US). Several 5-HT serotonin receptor agonists and antagonists are currently in the developing stages. Multiple classes of drugs are available for the symptomatic treatment of diarrhea and constipation, However, there is a need for more disease-specific agents.

Recommended reading

Bharucha AE, Dorn SD, Lembo A, Pressman A (2013) American Gastroenterological Association medical position statement on constipation. *Gastroenterology* Jan.; **144**(1): 211–17.

Brown, F, Drossman D, Gershon, M, *et al.* (2011) The tryptophan hydroxylase inhibitor LX1031 shows clinical benefit in patients with nonconstipating irritable bowel syndrome, *Gastroenterology* **141**: 507–16.

Camilleri M, Northcutt AR, Kong S, *et al.* (2000) Efficacy and safety of alosetron in women with irritable bowel syndrome: a randomised, placebo-controlled trial. *Lancet* **355**: 1035.

Camilleri M, Chey WY, Mayer EA, *et al.* (2001) A randomized controlled clinical trial of the serotonin type 3 receptor antagonist alosetron in women with diarrhea-predominant irritable bowel syndrome. *Arch Intern Med* **161**:1733.

Costedio MM, Hyman N, Mawe GM (2007) Serotonin and its role in colonic function and in gastrointestinal disorders, *Dis Colon and Rectum* **50**(3): 367–88.

Creed F, Fernandes L, Guthrie E, *et al.* (2003) The cost-effectiveness of psychotherapy and paroxetine for severe irritable bowel syndrome. *Gastroenterology* **124**: 303.

FDA. Drug information. www.fda.gov

Gershon MD, Tack J (2007) The serotonin signaling system: from basic understanding to drug development for functional GI disorders. *Gastroenterology* Jan.; **132**(1): 397–414.
Review of the role of the serotonin in the pathophysiology of functional bowel disorders.

Jones RH, Holtmann G, Rodrigo L, *et al.* (1999) Alosetron relieves pain and improves bowel function compared with mebeverine in female nonconstipated irritable bowel syndrome patients. *Aliment Pharmacol Ther* **13**: 1419.

Kellow J, Lee OY, Chang FY, *et al.* (2003) An Asia-Pacific, double blind, placebo controlled, randomized study to evaluate the efficacy, safety, and tolerability of tegaserod in patients with irritable bowel syndrome. *Gut* **52**: 671–6.

Tegaserod at 6 mg bid provided significant improvement in the global assessment of IBS symptoms and in individual symptoms, such as abdominal pain, bloating, and bowel habits, in 259 women with IBS-C when compared with placebo The primary efficacy variable (over weeks 1–4) was the response to the question: "Over the past week do you consider that you have had satisfactory relief from your IBS symptoms?" Secondary efficacy variables assessed overall satisfactory relief over 12 weeks and individual symptoms of IBS. Headache (12 % vs. 11.1% placebo) was the most common side effect.

Lexi-Comp, Inc. www.lexi.com

Li Z, Vaziri H (2012) Treatment of chronic diarrhea. *Best Pract Clin Gastroenterol* **26**(5): 677.

Tabas G, Beaves M, Wang J, Friday P, Mardini H, Arnold G (2004) Paroxetine to treat irritable bowel syndrome not responding to high-fiber diet: a double-blind, placebo-controlled trial. *Am J Gastroenterol* **99**(5): 914.

Tack J, Broekaert D, Fischler B, *et al.* (2006) A controlled crossover study of the selective serotonin reuptake inhibitor citalopram in irritable bowel syndrome. *Gut* **55**: 1095.

Vahedi H, Merat S, Rashidioon A, *et al.* (2005) The effect of fluoxetine in patients with pain and constipation-predominant irritable bowel syndrome: a double-blind randomized-controlled study. *Aliment Pharmacol Ther* **22**: 381.

Vazquez-Roque MI, Bouras EP (2013) Linaclotide, novel therapy for the treatment of chronic idiopathic constipation and constipation-predominant irritable bowel syndrome, *Adv Ther* Mar.; **30**(3): 203–11.

CHAPTER 6
5-aminosalicylates

Hannah L. Miller and Francis A. Farraye
Boston University School of Medicine, Boston, MA, USA

Introduction

The aminosalicylates are a class of drugs used as the initial treatment to induce and maintain remission in patients with mild to moderate ulcerative colitis (UC). Sulfasalazine (SASP) was first developed in the 1940s as a treatment for rheumatoid arthritis and was the first aminosalicylate to be used for the treatment of inflammatory bowel disease (IBD). However, as many as 20–25% of patients were found to be intolerant or allergic to sulfasalazine, and thus the 5-aminosalicylic acid (5-ASA) agents were developed. These medications encompass a wide variety of preparations, each with a 5-aminosalicylate moiety that is responsible for its anti-inflammatory activity. Unmodified 5-ASA is readily absorbed in the stomach and duodenum; thus modification of 5-ASA is needed to target release of the 5-ASA moiety at the site of active inflammation in the small bowel and colon.

Preparations

Many aminosalicylate preparations (oral or rectal administration) are approved for use in the United States, as well as other brands only available in Europe and Canada (Table 6.1). The 5-ASA family of medications includes: sulfasalazine (Azulfidine®), in which the 5-ASA is conjugated to sulfapyridine; mesalamine, in which the 5-ASA moiety is coated either with ethylcellulose (Pentasa®) or an acrylic-based resin, eudragit (Asacol HD®, Delzicol®); olsalazine (Dipentum®), in which two 5-ASA molecules are conjugated by an azo bond; and balsalazide (Colazal®, Giazo®), in which the 5-ASA moiety is conjugated to a 4-aminobenzoyl-beta-alanine carrier. Two once a day formulations of mesalamine are also available; one using a Multi-Matrix System (Lialda®) and the other with delayed release granules (Apriso®). Topical preparations of mesalamine are available in enema formulations (Rowasa®) as well as

Pocket Guide to Gastrointestinal Drugs, Edited by M. Michael Wolfe and Robert C. Lowe. © 2014 John Wiley & Sons, Ltd. Published 2014 by John Wiley & Sons, Ltd.

Table 6.1 Properties of oral 5-ASA preparations

Preparation	Products	Pill type	Solubility	Site of release	Pill specifications
Mesalamine coated with Eudragrit S	Asacol HD®	Tablet	pH >7	Distal ileum-colon	Do not crush
	Delzicol®	Capsule			Do not open
Mesalamine encapsulated in ethylcellulose microgranules	Pentasa®	Capsule	Time controlled release	Jejunum-ileum-colon	May open and place granules in apple sauce or yogurt
Mesalamine encapsulated in hydrophilic-lipophilic matrix	Lialda®	Tablet	pH>7	Colon	Do not crush
Mesalamine granules with coated with Eudragit L and polymer matrix core	Apriso®	Capsule	pH>6	Terminal ileum-colon	Do not open Off label: may open
Mesalamine coated with Eudragit L	Claversal®*	Tablet	pH >6	Jejunum-ileum-colon	Tablet: Do not crush or chew
	Mesasal®*	Tablet			Capsule: May open and consume granules
	Salofalk®*	Tablet or capsule			
Olsalazine (5-ASA + 5-ASA)	Dipentum®	Capsule	Colonic bacteria	Colon	May open
Balsalazide (4-aminobenzoyl-B-alanine + 5-ASA)	Colazal®	Capsule	Colonic bacteria	Colon	May open and sprinkle in applesauce, consume immediately
	Giazo®	Tablet			
Sulfasalazine (5-ASA + sulfapyridine)	Azulfidine®	Tablet	Colonic bacteria	Colon	Off label: oral suspension**

* Not available in the US.
**Compounding pharmacies can make oral suspensions of aminosalicylates; however, there are no pharmacokinetic studies ensuring adequate active drug levels are achieved.

suppositories (Canasa®). Outside the US, mesalamine is marketed under a variety of other brand names, including Salofalk®, Claversal®, Ipocal®, Mezavant®, Mezavant XL®, Mesacol®, VEGAZ_OD®, Mesacron®, and Mesalazina®. Asacol® standard release (400 mg tablet) is no longer available in the US due to an inactive ingredient in its enteric coating material, dibutyl phthalate (DBP), which at high doses in animal studies caused malformations. Asacol HD® (800 mg tablet) does contain DBP and remains available.

Clinical use and efficacy

The 5-aminosalicylates are approved for the treatment and mainte-nance of remission of ulcerative colitis in adults, with the exception of Apriso® and olsalazine, which are only approved for maintenance in UC (Table 6.2). Mesalamine has been shown to be very effective in the treatment of mild to moderate active UC. Seventy-two percent of patients receiving 4.8 g/day of mesalamine in the ASCEND II trial achieved treatment success, which was either complete remission or clinical response at week 6. The same study showed 4.8 g/day mesa-lamine was superior in achieving endoscopic and histologic remission in active UC, with 48% of patients achieving remission by sigmoido-scopic index ($p < 0.05$), compared with 31% on placebo, and 39% of patients achieving microscopic remission, compared with 23% on pla-cebo ($p < 0.03$). In the recent Cochrane meta-analysis, which include over 38 studies, there was no statistical difference in efficacy between once daily dosing 5-ASA and conventionally dosed 5-ASA. In addition when compared, 5-ASA was equal to sulfasalazine in inducing remis-sion in mild to moderate UC.

5-ASA has also been shown to be effective in maintaining remission of UC in randomized controlled trials, with 12-month remission rates of 64% (38% for placebo, $P = 0.0004$). In the recent Cochrane meta-analysis, 5-ASA was effective in maintenance of clinical and endoscopic remission with a relapse rate of 41% for 5-ASA patients compared with 58% for placebo (RR 0.69, 95% CI 0.62–0.77). Oral 5-ASA administered once daily was as effective as conventional dosing for maintenance of remission in quiescent UC. Sulfasalazine was found to be superior to 5-ASA for main-tenance of remission with 48% of 5-ASA patients relapsed compared to 43% of SASP patients (RR 1.14, 95% CI 1.03–1.27).

The 5-ASAs are not FDA approved for Crohn's disease (CD), and their role in induction and maintenance of remission in patients with CD remains controversial. CD clinical studies suffer from heteroge-neity of patients (disease locations, complications, previous surgery), varying doses of 5-ASA formulations, and primary endpoints using

Table 6.2 Commonly used 5-aminosalicylate drugs

Generic Name	Trade name	Adult dose	Common adult Rx	FDA indications	Off-label uses
Mesalamine	Delzicol®	400 mg capsule 1.6–2.4 g daily	2 capsules po tid on empty stomach^	Treatment and maintenance of mild-mod UC	Mild-mod Crohn's colitis
Measlamine	Asacol HD®	800 mg tablet 4.8 g daily	2 tablets po tid	Treatment of mild-mod UC*	Mild-mod Crohn's colitis
Mesalamine	Pentasa®	250 mg capsule 500 mg capsule 2–4 g daily	4 capsules po qid 2 capsules po qid	Treatment and maintenance of mild-mod UC	Mild-moderate Crohn's enteritis-colitis
Meslamine	Lialda®	1.2 g tablet 2.4–4.8 g daily	4 tablets po qd	Treatment and maintenance of mild-mod UC	Mild-mod Crohn's colitis
Mesalamine	Apriso®	0.375 mg capsule 1.5 g daily	4 capsules po daily	Maintenance of mild-mod UC**	Mild-mod Crohn's colitis
Balsalazide	Colazal®	750 mg capsule 6.75 g daily	3 capsules po tid	Treatment and maintenance mild-mod UC	Mild-mod Crohn's colitis
	Giazo®	1.1 gram tablet 6.6 g daily	3 tablets po bid	Treatment of mild-mod UC in male patients*	

(continued)

Table 6.2 (*Continued*)

Generic Name	Trade name	Adult dose	Common adult Rx	FDA indications	Off-label uses
Olsalazine	Dipentum®	500 mg capsule 2–3 g daily	2 capsules po tid	Maintenance of mild-mod UC**	Mild-mod Crohn's colitis
Sulfasalazine	Azulfidine®	500 mg capsule 3–6 g daily	Initial: 1 capsule po bid with meals, titrate every 3–5 days: 2 g, 3 g, 4 g to max 6 g if no clinical benefit Need: 1 mg/day folate	Treatment and maintenance of mild-mod UC Rheumatoid arthritis	Mild-mod Crohn's disease Ankylosing spondylitis Psoriasis
Mesalamine topical	Canasa®	1000 mg suppository	1000 mg pr qd	Treatment and maintenance of mild-mod UC proctitis	
Mesalamine topical	Rowasa®	4 g/60 ml enema	4 g pr qhs retain overnight	Treatment and maintenance of mild-mod distal UC	

*Drug is only approved for treatment (hasn't been studied beyond 8 weeks).
**Drug is only approved for maintenance.
^Manufacturer recommends 1 hour prior to food or 2 hours after food.

CDAI scores rather than endoscopic remission. In a pooled analysis of three clinical trials in active CD, Pentasa® 4 g/day was associated with a statistically significant reduction in CDAI compared to placebo (P = 0.04). Trials with other mesalamine formulations have shown between 45% to 55% clinical remission (CDAI<150), but none of them have used endoscopic remission as a primary endpoint. In the Cochrane meta-analysis, six RCTs examined the efficacy of 5-ASA in inducing remission in 910 active CD patients and found 68% randomized to 5-ASA did not achieve remission compared to 74% allocated to placebo, with a RR of 0.89 of not achieving remission with 5-ASA (95% CI = 0.80–0.99). This review also reported on two trials examining sulfasalazine in inducing remission in active CD and found 57% of patients randomized to sulfasalazine did not achieve remission compared with 68.9% for placebo, with a RR of 0.83 failure to achieve remission (95% CI = 0.69–1.00, p=0.05). Neither sulfasalazine nor mesalamine was effective in preventing relapse of CD. Despite this poor level of evidence, 5-ASA is commonly used off label for the treatment of Crohn's disease.

Pharmacology: preparations and dosing

Delayed-release mesalamine, Asacol HD® and Delzicol®, has an acid resistant acrylic resin that allows encapsulation of oral mesalamine, which releases the active drug when the luminal pH rises above 7 in the terminal ileum and colon (Table 6.1). Pentasa® has ethylcellulose microspheres that initiate the release of 5-ASA to the small intestine and colon. These two 5-ASA formulations are used off-label to treat Crohn's ileitis. Sulfasalazine, olsalazine, and balsalazide deliver 5-ASA predominately to the colon, since colonic bacteria are required to reduce the inactive parent drug to active 5-ASA in the colon. Both Lialda and Apriso have a pH-dependent release and thus target their release in the colon. All mesalamine preparations, including tablets, granules, and pellets, appear to be equally effective in inducing remission in active disease. Giazo was not found to be effective for women in clinical trials, and thus is approved for use only in men.

The American College of Gastroenterology (ACG) guidelines recommend combination oral and topical 5-ASA therapy for mild-to-moderate active left-sided or extensive UC disease. The dosage of oral mesalamine is between 2.4–4.8 g/day in divided doses. The optimal dose of oral mesalamine is controversial. The Cochrane meta-analysis showed no statistical significant difference in clinical improvement between mesalamine 4.8 g/day and 2.4 g/day, but subgroup analysis indicated that patients with moderate disease may benefit from the

Table 6.3 Pediatric dosing of 5-aminosalcylates

Generic name	Trade name	Pediatric dose
Mesalamine	Pentasa®	50–75 mg/kg/day divided in two to three doses max: 4 g/day

Balsalazide	Colazal®	Children 5–17 years:
		    2.25 g po TID (three 750 mg capsules TID)
		    or 750 mg po TID (one capsule TID)

Olsalazine	Dipentum®	25–35 mg/kg/day divided in two to three doses
Sulfasalazine	Azulfidine®	Mild: 40–50 mg/kg/day divided every 6 hours Mod-severe: 50–70 mg/kg/day divided every 4–6 hours, do not exceed 4 g/day Maintenance: 30–50 mg/kg/day divided every 4–8 hours, do not exceed 2 g/day
Mesalamine topical	Canasa®	1000 mg suppository pr qhs
Mesalamine topical	Rowasa®	4 g/60 ml enema pr qhs

Only sulfasalazine and balsalazide are FDA approved for pediatric ulcerative colitis.

higher dosing. Higher doses of mesalamine (4.8 g daily) have been shown to achieve higher rates of mucosal healing than lower doses. Most aminosalicylates can be started at their target doses with certain exceptions (Table 6.2 and 6.3). Sulfasalazine should be started gradually, and the dose increased as tolerated by 50–75 mg/kg per day to a target dose of 4–6 g/day. Patients should be supplemented with 1 mg folate daily while taking sulfasalazine. Clinical improvement is usually within 2–4 weeks.

For the maintenance of remission in distal UC, the ACG guidelines recommend topical mesalamine as an alternative to oral or combination therapy. Suppositories are used to treat proctitis up to 10 cm, while enemas can reach to the splenic flexure. In a meta-analysis of nine studies, rectal 5-ASA was effective for maintenance of both clinical and endoscopic remission over 6 months. The optimal dosing regimen of mesalamine suppositories and enemas has not been established, though studies have demonstrated that topical mesalamine preparations given as infrequently as three times weekly are effective in maintaining remission.

Mechanism of action

The specific mechanism responsible for the efficacy of 5-ASA compounds is unknown, although both anti-inflammatory and immunosupressive properties have been suggested *in vitro*. The anti-inflammatory properties include the ability of sulfasalazine and 5-ASA to inhibit cyclooxygenase and lipoxygenase, thereby inhibiting pro-inflammatory prostaglandins and leukotrienes. As a salicylic acid derivative, 5-ASA is also thought to have antioxidant properties that can decrease tissue injury. Furthermore, 5-ASA has also been shown to inhibit the activation of peripheral and intestinal lymphocytes, reduce leukocyte adhesion, and inhibit release of pro-inflammatory cytokines. Interleukin 1 (IL-1), tumor necrosis factor alpha, IL-2, IL-8, and NFκB are thought to be downregulated by 5-ASAs, thereby decreasing inflammation in intestinal mucosa. The immunosuppressive properties of 5-ASAs include the blockade of lymphocyte DNA synthesis and cell cycle progression and inhibition of T-cell proliferation, activation, and differentiation. The 5-ASAs are thought to possess antineoplastic (chemopreventive) properties as well.

Bioavailability and metabolism

The bioavailability and metabolism of each 5-ASA compound is dependent on its pharmacology (Table 6.4). Pharmacokinetic profiles of the 5-ASA formulations show comparable systemic absorption for pH-dependent, controlled release, and prodrug formulations. The different types of delivery systems do not affect the clinical response to 5-ASA drugs.

Approximately 28% of mesalamine is absorbed after oral ingestion, leaving the remainder available for topical mucosal activity, which is excreted in the feces. The small portion of absorbed mesalamine is rapidly acetylated in the gut mucosal wall and by the liver, and then excreted by the kidneys as N-acetyl-5-aminosalicylic acid. Absorption of mesalamine is similar in fasted and fed subjects. Sulfasalazine is partially absorbed in the jejunum after oral ingestion. The remainder passes into the colon, where it is reduced by bacterial enzyme azoreductase to sulfapyridine and 5-ASA. Following absorption, sulfapyridine undergoes acetylation to form AcSP and ring hydroxylation. Most of the absorbed sulfasalazine is excreted into bile, with only a minority excreted in the urine. The sulfapyridine component is absorbed from the colon, metabolized in the liver and excreted mostly in the urine, and only a small portion remains in the feces. 5-ASA undergoes N-acetylation, and the rate of metabolism via acetylation is dependent upon patient's acetylation phenotype.

Pharmacokinetic data show the amount of absorbed mesalamine is different among these drugs. Delayed-release mesalamine appears to be

Table 6.4 Bioavailability and metabolism

Drug	Absorption	Metabolism	Half-life	Time to peak, serum	Elimination
Sulfasalazine	<15% parent drug in small bowel	Colonic bacteria 5-ASA portion: liver and intestine	Dependent on acetylator phenotype: Fast: 5.7–10 hrs Slow: 14.8 hrs	3–12 hours metabolites: 10 hours	Primarily urine
Mesalamine	Tablet: 20–28% Capsule: 20–40%	Liver and intestine	5-ASA: 0.5–10 hrs N-acetyl-5-ASA: 2–15 hours	AsacolHD® and Delzicol®. 4–12 hours Lialda®: 9–12 hours Apriso®: 4 hours Pentasa®: 3 hours	Urine (primarily metabolites) <8% unchanged drug <2% feces
Balsalazide	Minimal	Azo reduced by colonic bacteria	No systemic half life	1–2 hours	Feces (65% as 5-ASA and other metabolites) Urine (<16% as N-acetylated metabolite) <1% of parent drug is seen
Olsalazine	<3% very little systemically absorbed	Colonic bacteria 0.1%metabolized by liver	54 minutes	1 hour	Primarily feces <1% urine

more extensively absorbed than the mesalamine released from sulfasalazine. Plasma levels of mesalamine and N-acetyl-5-minosalicylic acid are 1.5–2 times higher than those following equivalent dose of mesalamine in the form of sulfasalazine. Four grams of sulfasalazine provides 1.6 grams of mesalamine to the colon. This plasma level difference does not appear to translate into a difference in the clinical response. The delayed-release mesalamine products have not been shown to be bioequivalent according to the manufacturer (two Delzicol® capsules and one Asacol HD® tablet).

The extent of absorption of Rowasa® enema is dependent upon the retention time of the drug. At steady state, approximately 10–30% of the daily 4 gram dose can be recovered in cumulative 24 hour urine collections. Bioavailability characteristics of absorbed mesalamine and other organ distribution are not known. Mesalamine administered as a rectal suppository is variably absorbed. Rectal tissue concentrations for 5-ASA and N-acetyl-5-ASA have not been systematically quantified. In UC patients treated with mesalamine 500 mg rectal suppositories once every eight hours (more frequent than clinical practice) for six days, the mean mesalamine peak plasma concentration was 361 ng/mL at steady state.

Adverse effects and toxicity

As a class of agents, 5-aminosalicylates are generally well-tolerated (Table 6.5). Based on RCT data, the estimate of all adverse events is between 20 and 30%, with the most common side effects being mild in severity including headache, nausea, worsening diarrhea, and a withdrawal rate of 5–10%. Mesalamine has been implicated in the production of acute intolerance syndrome, characterized by acute abdominal pain, bloody diarrhea, fever, headache, and rash which occurred in 3% of patients treated with mesalamine delayed-release tablets in controlled clinical trials. Olsalazine may cause a worsening of diarrhea by enhancing bicarbonate secretion in the small intestine, which increases fluid volumes delivered to the colon. Rowasa enemas have very few side effects, with low rates of abdominal pain, cramping, flatulence, and headache. Canasa, suppositories are very well-tolerated, with the most common side effect, dizziness, seen in 3% of patients.

Intolerance to sulfasalazine, characterized by headache, nausea, vomiting, anorexia, and myalgias, is managed by lowering the dose and titrating slowly to therapeutic range, and it is often seen in phenotypically slow acetylators. Sulfasalazine and rarely other 5-ASAs can cause a hypersensitivity reaction, ranging from fever and rash to more generalized allergic reactions. Bone marrow suppression with leukopenia, and rarely agranulocytosis, occurs and can be managed by dose reduction or discontinuation. Frequent blood monitoring is recommended by the

Table 6.5 Adverse effects and toxicity of 5-aminosalicylates

Drug	Common >10%	Uncommon 1-10%	Rare <1%
Sulfasalazine	Headache Rash Nausea, vomiting Anorexia Dyspepsia Oligospermia (reversible)	Pancreatitis Fever Stomatitis Urticaria Hemolytic anemia Leukopenia	Pneumonitis Agranulocytosis Otalgia Alopecia Hepatitis
Mesalamine	Headache Eructation/ belching	Nausea Diarrhea Rash Fever Pharyngitis Tinnitus	Pericarditis Nephritis Pneumonitis Thrombocytopenia Pancreatitis Hepatitis Alopecia
Olsalazide	Watery Diarrhea	Abdominal cramps Nausea Arthralgias	Pericarditis Nephritis Pneumonitis Thrombocytopenia Pancreatitis Hepatitis Alopecia Stomatitis
Balsalazide	Headache	Fever Abdominal pain Diarrhea Arthralgia Nausea Stomatitis	Pericarditis Nephritis Pneumonitis Thrombocytopenia Pancreatitis Hepatitis Alopecia

manufacturer (Table 6.6). Sulfasalazine is associated with the development of oligospermia and reduced sperm motility, which is due to the sulfapyridine moiety. This male infertility is reversible with drug discontinuation.

Several serious adverse events have been reported in case reports, including interstitial nephritis, pneumonitis, and pancreatitis, which are all reversible with cessation of the drug. The pathogenesis of interstitial nephritis is unknown; however, it may be due to intra-renal prostaglandin dysregulation. Reassuringly, the risk of chronic renal injury is low if the diagnosis is made and therapy stopped within

Table 6.6 Monitoring recommendations while on 5-aminosalicylates

	Initial labs	Future labs*
Sulfasalazine	CBC with diff and liver function tests	CBC with diff and liver function tests every other week × 3 months, monthly × 3 months, and then q3 months Urinalysis and renal function periodically
5-aminosalicylates	Creatinine CBC (in elderly)	Creatinine periodically CBC periodically

*Recommended by manufacturer.

10 months. Periodic evaluation of renal function is recommended (Table 6.6). Acute pancreatitis has been described in patients with both sulfasalazine and mesalamine, using both oral and rectal formulations. This adverse effect has been seen both after prolonged therapy duration and with re-challenge. Although pancreatitis is considered an extra-intestinal manifestation of IBD, epidemiologic evidence suggests that mesalamine users have a higher rate of pancreatitis. The mechanism is thought to be via free radical generation causing direct tissue damage in the pancreas.

Pregnancy (Table 6.7)

Sulfasalazine, Delzicol®, Pentasa®, Apriso®, Lialda®, and balsalazide are considered safe agents in pregnancy, with an FDA category B. Asacol HD remains a category C and should only be used in pregnancy if clearly needed, according to the manufacturer. There has been no reports fetal malformations in women taking mesalamine during pregnancy. Although early cohort studies showed increased preterm deliveries and stillbirth, this adverse effect has been attributed to disease activity and not to 5-ASA. Olsalazine is considered FDA category C as it has been shown to produce fetal developmental toxicity (reduced fetal weights, retarded ossifications, and immaturity of the fetal visceral organs) when given during organogenesis to pregnant rats in doses 5–20 times the human dose (100–400 mg/kg). There are no adequate and well-controlled studies in pregnant women. Olsalazine should be used during pregnancy only if the potential benefit justifies the potential risk to the fetus, according to the manufacturer.

Table 6.7 Pregnancy and lactation for 5-aminosalicylates

	Pregnancy	Lactation	Breast feeding effect seen in newborn
Sulfasalazine	Category B	Enters breast milk Use with caution	Kernicterus
Asacol HD®	Category C	Enters breast milk Use with caution	Diarrhea
Delzicol®	Category B		
Apriso®	Category B		
Pentasa®	Category B		
Lialda®	Category B		
Olsalazide	Category C	Enters breast milk Not recommended	Diarrhea
Balsalzide	Category B	Excretion in breast milk unknown Use with caution	Bloody diarrhea

Drug interactions (package inserts)

Because the dissolution of the coating of mesalamine granules is pH-dependent, mesalamine sustained release products, i.e Apriso®, Lialda®, Asacol HD®, and Delzicol®, should not be co-administered with antacids, H_2-antagonists, and proton pump inhibitors. Separating administration time between mesalamine and antacids may be adequate to avoid this interaction. 5-ASA derivatives may decrease serum concentration of cardiac glycosides (digoxin), and monitoring is thus advised. The co-administration of 5-ASA agents with 6-mercaptopurine or azathioprine may result in an increased risk of myelosuppression, and monitoring white blood cell count is accordingly recommended when 5-ASAs are added or withdrawn in patients on these agents. It is recommended not to give salicylates for six weeks after the varicella vaccine to avoid a possible increased risk of developing Reye's syndrome.

Precautions and contraindications (Table 6.8)

Aminosalicylates are contraindicated in patients with hypersensitivity to salicylates or to any of the components of the tablets. Patients with an allergy to any of the compounds used to make the drug products must avoid use, including those allergic to phenylalanine in

Table 6.8 Contraindications and precautions of 5-aminosalicylates

	Contraindications	Warning/precaution	Special considerations
Sulfasalazine	Sulfonamide allergy: hypersensitivity to sulfa or salicylates Porphyria GI or GU obstruction	Cross reaction in allergies to loop and thiazide diuretics G6PD deficiency Blood dyscrasias Folate deficiency Caution in renal and liver impairment	Slow acetylators: prolonged half-life of sulfapyrazine metabolite
Mesalamine	Hypersensitivity to mesalamine or salicylates		Elderly: increase blood dyscrasias Delayed gastric emptying (pyloric stenosis): retention of tablets will delay release of mesalamine in colon
Olsalazide	Hypersensitivity to olsalazine or salicylates	Diarrhea may worsen	
Balsalazide	Hypersensitivity to balsazide metabolites or salicylates	Diarrhea may worsen	Teeth staining if capsule opened and consume granules

Apriso®, saturated vegetable fatty acid esters in the Canasa® suppository vehicle, and potassium metabisulfite (sulfite) in the suspension formula of Rowasa®.

Most patients who develop an allergic reaction to sulfasalazine can tolerate the 5-ASAs because the allergy is most commonly due to the sulfa moiety. Sulfasalazine should be given with caution to patients with severe allergy or bronchial asthma. Chemical similarities are present among sulfonamides, sulfonylureas, carbonic anhydrase inhibitors, thiazides, and loop diuretics; therefore, a risk of cross-reaction exists in patients with allergy to any of these compounds. Adequate fluid intake must be maintained in order to prevent crystalluria and stone formation. Patients with glucose-6 phosphate dehydrogenase deficiency should be observed closely for signs of hemolytic anemia. This reaction is frequently dose related.

Caution should be advised when administering aminosalicylates to patients with liver or renal disease. There have been reports of hepatic failure in patients with pre-existing liver disease. Renal impairment, including minimal change nephropathy, acute and chronic interstitial nephritis, and renal failure, has been reported when mesalamine was administered to patients with renal dysfunction. Periodic blood monitoring is recommended (Table 6.6).

Special considerations: effectiveness in colorectal cancer prevention

Multiple studies have assessed the utility of 5-ASA in preventing dysplasia and cancer in patients with UC. These results have differed depending on the type of population in the study, whether referral based, nonreferral, or clinic-based populations. The meta-analysis suggesting a chemopreventive effect was by Velayos *et al.* and included 9 observational studies involving 1932 patients with UC. This study reported a positive association between 5-ASA use and colorectal cancer (CRC) (OR 0.51; 95% CI: 0.37–0.69) or a combined endpoint of CRC and dysplasia (OR 0.51; 95% CI: 0.38–0.69), which equates to a 49% reduction in the risk of CRC or CRC/dysplasia with regular 5-ASA use. The optimal dose of 5-ASA for chemoprevention is thought to be at least 1.2 grams/day of mesalamine, which provided the greatest dose reduction of 72%–81%.

In contrast, a recent Cochrane meta-analysis of nonreferral populations included four studies with over 608 cases and 2177 controls found no protective effect of 5-ASA on CRC in IBD, with pooled adjusted OR 0.95 (95% CI: 0.66–1.38). The authors also examined a separate meta-analysis of nine clinic-based studies, which in contrast yielded a pooled OR of 0.58 (95% CI: 0.45–0.75), although noting that a wide heterogeneity among the studies limits their interpretation. Issues with these meta-analyses are considerable. For example, different dosages of 5-ASA were used; some included sulfasalazine while others did not, and a wide variation of time intervals of exposure to 5-ASA prior to cancer detection was used (i.e., only 3 months compared with others that used years). Results also widely vary depending on the geographic location in the world, as some areas have higher rates of CRC and on the, study populations that incorporated an older patient, as these cohort would have higher rates of cancer as well.

Table 6.9 Summary of 5-Aminosalicylates

Products	Site of release	Mg	Dosing
Asacol HD® Delzicol®	Distal ileum-colon	800 mg 400 mg	2 tablets tid 2 capsules tid*
Pentasa®	Jejunum-ileum-colon	250 mg 500 mg	4 capsules qid 2 capsules qid
Lialda®	Colon	1.2 mg	4 tablets qd
Apriso®	Terminal ileum-colon	0.375 mg	4 capsules qd
Dipentum®	Colon	500 mg	2 capsules tid
Colazal® Giazo®**	Colon	750 mg 1.1 g	3 capsules tid 3 tablets bid
Azulfidine®	Colon	500 mg	1 capsule bid, titrate up to 4–6 g/day
Rowasa®	Rectum	4 g/60 ml	Enema PR qhs Retain overnight
Canasa®	Rectum	1000 mg	1 PR qhs

*Administered without food (1 hour prior to food or 2 hours after food).
**Only approved for use in men.

Conclusion (Table 6.9)

The 5-aminosalycilate class of medications is highly effective in inducing and maintaining remission in 40–80% of UC patients, with equal efficacy among the different agents. Many different preparations exist. In addition, the excellent safety profile of aminosalicylates make them first line treatment for mild to moderate UC.

Recommended reading

Asacol (package insert) (2011) Rockaway, NJ: Warner Chilcott LLC.
Azulfidine (package insert) (2011) New York, NY Pfizer Inc.
Bantel H, Berg C, Vieth M, Stolte M, Kruis W, Schulze-Osthoff K (2000) Mesalazine inhibits activation of transcription factor NF-kappaB in inflamed mucosa of patients with ulcerative colitis. *Gastroenterology* **95**(12): 3452–7. Epub 2001/01/11.
Canasa (package insert) (2008) Birmingham, AL: Axcan Pharma US, Inc.
Delzicol (package insert) (2013) Germany: Warner Chilcott Deutschland GmbH.
Feagan BG, Macdonald JK (2012a) Oral 5-aminosalicylic acid for induction of remission in ulcerative colitis. *Cochrane Database Syst Rev* **10**: CD000543. Epub 2012/10/19.

This meta-analysis shows that 5-ASA is superior to placebo but no more effective than sulfasalazine in inducing remission of UC and patients with moderate disease may benefit from higher 4.8 g/day dosing.

Feagan BG, Macdonald JK (2012b) Oral 5-aminosalicylic acid for maintenance of remission in ulcerative colitis. *Cochrane Database Syst Rev* **10**: CD000544. Epub 2012/10/19.

This meta-analysis compares the efficacy of oral 5-ASA administered once daily which is as effective as conventional dosing for maintenance of remission in UC, and also demonstrates 5-ASA has a statistically significant therapeutic inferiority relative to sulfasalazine.

Fernandez J, Sala M, Panes J, Feu F, Navarro S, Teres J (1997) Acute pancreatitis after long-term 5-aminosalicylic acid therapy. *Gastroenterology* **92**(12): 2302–3. Epub 1997/12/17.

Ford AC, Kane SV, Khan KJ, Achkar JP, Talley NJ, Marshall JK, *et al.* (2011) Efficacy of 5-aminosalicylates in Crohn's disease: systematic review and meta-analysis. *Gastroenterology* **106**(4): 617–29. Epub 2011/03/17.

Ford AC, Khan KJ, Achkar JP, Moayyedi P (2012) Efficacy of oral vs. topical, or combined oral and topical 5-aminosalicylates, in ulcerative colitis: systematic review and meta-analysis. *Gastroenterology* **107**(2): 167–76; author reply 77. Epub 2011/11/24.

Giazo (package insert) (2012) Morrisville, NC: Salix Pharmaceuticals.

Hanauer SB, Stromberg U (2004) Oral Pentasa in the treatment of active Crohn's disease: A meta-analysis of double-blind, placebo-controlled trials. *Clinical Gastroenterology and Hepatology: The Official Clinical Practice Journal of the American Gastroenterological Association* **2**(5): 379–88. Epub 2004/05/01.

Hanauer S, Schwartz J, Robinson M, Roufail W, Arora S, Cello J, *et al.* (1993) Mesalamine capsules for treatment of active ulcerative colitis: results of a controlled trial. Pentasa Study Group. *Gastroenterology* **88**(8): 1188–97. Epub 1993/08/01.

Hanauer SB, Sandborn WJ, Kornbluth A, Katz S, Safdi M, Woogen S, *et al.* (2005) Delayed-release oral mesalamine at 4.8 g/day (800 mg tablet) for the treatment of moderately active ulcerative colitis: the ASCEND II trial. *Gastroenterology* **100**(11): 2478–85. Epub 2005/11/11.

Kornbluth A, Sachar DB (2010) Ulcerative colitis practice guidelines in adults: American College Of Gastroenterology, Practice Parameters Committee. *Gastroenterology* **105**(3): 501–23; quiz 24. Epub 2010/01/14.

Kruis W, Bar-Meir S, Feher J, Mickisch O, Mlitz H, Faszczyk M, *et al.* (2003) The optimal dose of 5-aminosalicylic acid in active ulcerative colitis: a dose-finding study with newly developed mesalamine. *Clinical Gastroenterology and Hepatology: The Official Clinical Practice Journal of the American Gastroenterological Association* **1**(1): 36–43. Epub 2004/03/16.

Lichtenstein GR, Ramsey D, Rubin DT (2011) Randomised clinical trial: delayed-release oral mesalazine 4.8 g/day vs. 2.4 g/day in endoscopic mucosal healing – ASCEND I and II combined analysis. *Alimentary Pharmacology and Therapeutics*. **33**(6): 672–8. Epub 2011/01/25.

This landmark randomized clinical trial showed 4.8g/day mesalamine achieves higher mucosal healing than 2.4g/day in active ulcerative colitis

Mahadevan U, Kane S (2006) American gastroenterological association institute technical review on the use of gastrointestinal medications in pregnancy. *Gastroenterology* **131**(1): 283–311. Epub 2006/07/13.

Marshall JK, Thabane M, Steinhart AH, Newman JR, Anand A, Irvine EJ (2012) Rectal 5-aminosalicylic acid for maintenance of remission in ulcerative colitis. *Cochrane Database Syst Rev* **11**: CD004118. Epub 2012/11/16.
This is the recent meta-analysis concluding that rectal 5-ASA is effective in maintaining remission of mild to moderate distal UC, both clinical as well as endoscopic.

Miner P, Hanauer S, Robinson M, Schwartz J, Arora S (1995) Safety and efficacy of controlled-release mesalamine for maintenance of remission in ulcerative colitis. Pentasa UC Maintenance Study Group. *Digestive Diseases and Sciences* **40**(2): 296–304. Epub 1995/02/01.

Moss AC, Peppercorn MA (2007) The risks and the benefits of mesalazine as a treatment for ulcerative colitis. *Expert Opinion on Drug Safety* **6**(2): 99–107. Epub 2007/03/21.

Nguyen GC, Gulamhusein A, Bernstein CN (2012) 5-aminosalicylic acid is not protective against colorectal cancer in inflammatory bowel disease: a meta-analysis of non-referral populations. *Gastroenterology* **107**(9): 1298–1304. Epub 2012/07/04.

Rowasa (package insert) (2008) Marietta, GA: Alaven Pharmaceuticals LLC.

Rubin DT, LoSavio A, Yadron N, Huo D, Hanauer SB (2006) Aminosalicylate therapy in the prevention of dysplasia and colorectal cancer in ulcerative colitis. *Clinical Gastroenterology and Hepatology: The Official Clinical Practice Journal of the American Gastroenterological Association* **4**(11): 1346–50. Epub 2006/10/25.

Saez J, Martinez J, Garcia C, Grino P, Perez-Mateo M (2000) Idiopathic pancreatitis associated with ulcerative colitis. *Gastroenterology* **95**(10): 3004–5. Epub 2000/10/29.

Sandborn WJ, Hanauer SB (2003) Systematic review: the pharmacokinetic profiles of oral mesalazine formulations and mesalazine pro-drugs used in the management of ulcerative colitis. *Alimentary Pharmacology & Therapeutics* **17**(1): 29–42. Epub 2002/12/21.

Sandborn WJ, Regula J, Feagan BG, Belousova E, Jojic N, Lukas M, *et al.* (2009) Delayed-release oral mesalamine 4.8 g/day (800-mg tablet) is effective for patients with moderately active ulcerative colitis. *Gastroenterology* **137**(6): 1934–43 e1-3. Epub 2009/09/22.

Shanahan F, Niederlehner A, Carramanzana N, Anton P (1990) Sulfasalazine inhibits the binding of TNF alpha to its receptor. *Immunopharmacology* **20**(3): 217–24. Epub 1990/11/01.

Stevens C, Lipman M, Fabry S, Moscovitch-Lopatin M, Almawi W, Keresztes S, *et al.* (1995) 5-Aminosalicylic acid abrogates T-cell proliferation by blocking interleukin-2 production in peripheral blood mononuclear cells. *Journal of Pharmacology and Experimental Therapeutics* **272**(1): 399–406. Epub 1995/01/01.

Velayos FS, Terdiman JP, Walsh JM (2005) Effect of 5-aminosalicylate use on colorectal cancer and dysplasia risk: a systematic review and metaanalysis of observational studies. *Gastroenterology* **100**(6): 1345–53. Epub 2005/06/03.
This meta-analysis was the key paper that showed a protective association between 5-aminosalicylates and colorectal cancer in patients with ulcerative colitis.

World MJ, Stevens PE, Ashton MA, Rainford DJ (1996) Mesalazine-associated interstitial nephritis. *Nephrology, Dialysis, Transplantation* **11**(4): 614–21. Epub 1996/04/01.

CHAPTER 7

Immunosuppressive agents

Lev Lichtenstein and Gerald M. Fraser

Rabin Medical Center, Beilinson Hospital, Petah Tikva, Israel

Introduction

Immunosuppressive agents or immunomodulators are general terms referring to drugs used to modulate and inhibit the activity of the immune system. The three main categories of immunomodulators used for the treatment of gastrointestinal diseases are thiopurines, methotrexate and calcineurin inhibitors.

Initially intended mainly for transplant medicine, immunomodulators have proven efficacy in numerous chronic inflammatory conditions and their use in inflammatory bowel disease, while never formally approved, is widely endorsed by professional organizations and have become a cornerstone of the treatment algorithms.

The main uses of immunomodulators in *inflammatory bowel disease* are:

- induction of clinical remission (methotrexate, cyclosporine (CsA));
- prevention of inflammatory relapses (thiopurines, methotrexate);
- support of tapering down corticosteroids (steroid-sparing effect, thiopurines, methotrexate); and
- prevention of immune neutralization of biological treatment (thiopurines, methotrexate).

In addition, thiopurines and cyclosporine are effective in the treatment of *autoimmune hepatitis.*

Thiopurines

Introduction of drug class

Azathioprine (AZA) and the closely related 6-mercaptopurine (6-MP) and 6-thioguanine (6-TG) are immunosuppressive drugs that belong to the chemical class of purine analogs. These drugs have proven efficacy and are extensively used for maintenance of remission in Crohn's

Pocket Guide to Gastrointestinal Drugs, Edited by M. Michael Wolfe and Robert C. Lowe. © 2014 John Wiley & Sons, Ltd. Published 2014 by John Wiley & Sons, Ltd.

disease and ulcerative colitis; approximately four patients would need to be treated to prevent relapse in one. They are used for the prevention of postoperative recurrence in Crohn's patients. Their co-administration with biological therapy and steroid sparing represent other recommended off-label applications

Basic pharmacology
Mechanisms of action
Thiopurine metabolites are structurally similar to purine nucleic acids. Intermediate metabolites enter purine enzymatic pathways, compete with purines and interfere with the synthesis of purine nucleotides. By incorporation into DNA, the thiopurine end-metabolite 6-thioguanine nucleotide (6-TGN) induces apoptosis of actively proliferating immune cells. While the effect on clonal expansion of lymphocytes is not sufficient to terminate the acute inflammatory process, depletion of antigen-specific memory T-cells effectively prevents further relapses of inflammation

Bioavailability
AZA is well-absorbed, but the bioavailability of 6MP is relatively limited (~50%).

Metabolism (Figure 7.1)
AZA is quickly and nonenzymatically cleaved to 6-MP.
Further metabolism occurs by three competing pathways:
1 Conversion by hypoxanthine phosphoribosyltransferase (HPRT) into 6-thioinosine 5′-monophosphate (6-TiMP), which is further metabolized to active 6-thioguanine nucleotides (6-TGN) and 6-MMP ribonucleotides (6-MMPR).

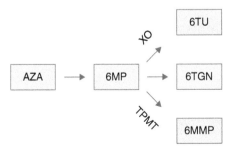

Figure 7.1 Metabolism of thiopurines. 6-MMP: 6-methylmercaptopurine; 6-MP, 6-mercaptopurine; 6-TGN: thioguanine nucleotide; 6-TU, thiouric acid; AZA, azathioprine; TPMT, thiopurine methyltransferase; XO: xanthine oxidase.

2 Methylation by thiopurine methyltransferase (TPMT) into an inactive 6-methyl-mercaptopurine (6-MMP). Exaggerated activity of this pathway in "rapid methylators" leads to accumulation of potentially hepatotoxic 6-MMP; resulting elevation of liver enzymes might require discontinuation of the drug.

3 Oxidation by xanthine oxidase (XO) into an inactive 6-thiouric acid (6-TU). This inducible degradation pathway may take several weeks to reach its maximal activity.

Genetic polymorphism in the TPMT gene makes TPMT activity highly variable

Approximately 0.3% of the population possesses a pair of nonfunctional alleles. Resulting absent TPMT activity renders such patients, if commenced on thiopurines, susceptible to severe and life-threatening myelotoxicity. Another 11% of individuals inherit one functional and one nonfunctional allele (heterozygous), conferring intermediate TPMT activity. The remaining 89% are homozygous for the allele conferring normal activity. Pre-treatment assessment of TPMT status (by geno- or phenotyping) is generally advised and can help to identify patients at risk for severe myelosuppression.

Metabolite monitoring

Assessment of metabolite levels can help to predict the likelihood of both the clinical efficacy and the myelo- and hepatotoxicity (Table 7.1).

Special safety concerns

The antigout compound *allopurinol* effectively blocks xanthine oxidase (XO) purine degradation pathway, shifting thiopurine metabolite flow into the unaffected methylation and 6-TGN-producing trails. The methylation pathway eventually becomes saturated, rending most of the thiopurine into the 6-TGN-producing trail and resulting in rapid and severe myelosuppression. *In general, the two drugs should not be administered together.*

Occasionally, exaggerated methylation activity ("rapid methylators") results in the accumulation of hepatotoxic 6-MMP and does not

Table 7.1 Assessment of metabolite levels		
6-Thioguanine [6-TG]	$> 230 \, \text{pmol}/8 \times 10^8 \, \text{RBC}$	Clinical efficacy
6-Methylmercaptopurine [6-MMP]	$> 5700 \, \text{pmol}/8 \times 10^8 \, \text{RBC}$	Hepatotoxicity

permit adequate dosing of thiopurines. In selected cases, allocation of the metabolite flow to 6-TGN by cautious co-administration of allopurinol enables substantial reduction of the required AZA/6MP dose, indirectly helping to restore tolerable levels of 6-MMP. Such concomitant treatment requires meticulous monitoring of 6-TG, however safety concerns remain.

Main drug interaction
Drugs that interfere with the metabolism of thiopurines and potentially myelosuppressive agents should be used with caution (Table 7.2).

Adverse effects
Tolerability issues are not infrequent and may limit treatment in up to 20% of the patients.

Adverse effects can be divided into three major categories:
- gastrointestinal intolerance;
- idiosyncratic (including allergic) reactions;
- pharmacologically explainable dose-dependent effects.

The potential risk of infection and neoplastic complications represent additional concerns of chronic immunosuppression.

Gastrointestinal intolerance
Nausea and vomiting are reported by up to 10% of the patients, most often during the first weeks of the treatment, and comprise the major obstacle to patient adherence. These symptoms can be minimized by gradually increasing the dose and administration with meals. Split-dose administration may represent an alternative option. Substituting 6-MP for AZA may also be helpful in some. Blood work to exclude possibility of allergic pancreatitis is mandatory.

Table 7.2 Drugs that interfere with the metabolism of thiopurines and potentially myelosuppressive agents

Drug	Interaction	Effect	Comment
Allopurinol	Inhibit XO	$\uparrow\uparrow\uparrow$6TG	Undesirable
Aminosalicylates	Inhibit TPMT	$\uparrow$6TG	Favorable clinical response
Infliximab	?	$\uparrow$6TG	
Sulfamethoxazole-trimethoprim Ribavirin ACE inhibitors	Potentiate myelosuppressive properties of thiopurines		Use with caution

Idiosyncratic reactions and hypersensitivity

Fever, rashes, muscle and joint pains are reported in up to 5% of patients and usually represent hypersensitivity to the imidazolyl (rather than mercaptopurine) moiety of AZA. These symptoms may not necessarily recur upon re-challenge with 6-MP.

In contrast, allergic pancreatitis (1%) results from hypersensitivity to the mercaptopurine portion of the AZA molecule and practically precludes switching to 6-MP. Treatment with 6-thioguanine can be considered as an alternative for those who are allergic to AZA/6-MP. Specific side effects such as nodular regenerative hyperplasia limit extensive use of this medication.

Dose-dependent effects

Myelotoxicity

The most significant toxic effect of thiopurines is myelosuppression, which should be anticipated in up to 2% of the patients. If this adverse effect occurs early in treatment, myelosuppression might indicate non-functional alleles of TPMT. Delayed myelosuppression is usually related to unforeseen drug interactions or temporary immunosuppression by intercurrent viral infections

Careful monitoring of blood counts is mandatory. Pre-treatment TPMT testing cannot substitute for regular blood work (Table 7.3).

Evidence of modest myelosuppression (WBC $< 4 \times 10^9$/L or platelet $< 120 \times 10^9$/L) warrants dose adjustment; profound drop of the counts prompts temporary discontinuation of the treatment.

Macrocytosis

Elevation of mean corpuscular volume (MCV) of red blood cells is frequently observed and, after other possible causes excluded, can actually indicate compliance with the treatment.

Table 7.3 Monitoring of blood counts	
	Required frequency of CBC test
First 4 weeks (or after dose escalation)	On a weekly basis
2nd and 3rd months	Bi-weekly
4th-6th months	Monthly
Then (on stable dose)	Every 3 months

Elevated liver enzymes
Methylation is a main metabolic pathway of thiopurines during the first weeks of the treatment and leads to temporary elevation of hepatotoxic 6-MMP levels. Mild and transient elevation of liver transaminases is frequently (13%) observed and does not necessarily signal a chronic, serious liver problem. Temporary adjustment of the dose to allow adequate time for induction of oxidation metabolic pathways is usually sufficient. In contrast, a rapid and steep (X4) elevation of GGT might indicate clinically significant hepatotoxicity and warrants prompt discontinuation of the treatment. Serious problems such as mercaptopurine moiety-related cholestasis, veno-occlusive disease and nodular regenerative hyperplasia are extremely rare.

Infection
Infections are a constant concern for patients receiving chronic immunosuppression. With this concern in mind, it should be noted that treatment of IBD patients with thiopurines has not been associated with the risk of serious infection. There is also no evidence for a diminished immune response to vaccination.

Association with neoplasia
Lymphoproliferative disorders
Chronic immunosuppression results in defective T-cell immunosurveillance, raising a concern of potential development of *lymphoproliferative disorders*. Thiopurines have been reported to increase the risk of lymphoma up to five-fold, yet the absolute risk appears to be quite low.

Hepatosplenic T-cell lymphoma (HSTCL)
HSTCL is an extremely rare and very aggressive lymphoproliferative disorder reported in IBD patients treated with thiopurines, with or without concomitant treatment with a TNFα antagonist.

Nonmelanoma skin cancer
The use of thiopurines is associated with an increased risk of nonmelanoma skin cancer in IBD patients. Periodic examination by a dermatologist and appropriate sun protection are advised.

Dosing information (Table 7.4)
The optimal protocol for introducing treatment with thiopurines has not been established. Most experts advocate a low starting dose, with subsequent titration of the dose according to clinical response and adverse events; some use decreased daily doses in TPMT heterozygotes.

Table 7.4 Dosing information		
Drug	**Initial dose**	**Maximum daily dose**
AZA	0.5–1.5 mg/kg	2.0–3.0 mg/kg
6MP	0.25–0.5 mg/kg	1.0–1.5 mg/kg

Tailoring dose adjustment according to levels of 6-TG and 6-MMP metabolites is another possible strategy. It should be stressed that none of these strategies replaces proper monitoring of blood counts and liver enzymes.

Pregnancy considerations

FDA designates thiopurines as Category D. In a large meta-analysis of patients with IBD, early exposure to thiopurines was associated with preterm birth. A possible association with congenital abnormalities, low birth weight, or spontaneous abortions was suggested in the past yet was not confirmed by recent large studies. The expert consensus is that in patients responding to thiopurines, the clinical benefit of the treatment usually outweighs the potential risks to the fetus.

Breastfeeding

Thiopurines and metabolites are detectable in breast milk, yet at very low levels. Breastfed neonates show no signs of immunosuppression. Thus, women receiving thiopurines need not be discouraged from breastfeeding.

Administration in children

Both North American and European Pediatric Gastroenterology Societies endorse the use of thiopurines.

Administration in hepatic or renal impairment

The treatment is safe in patients with impaired renal function; no dose reduction required. Careful monitoring of blood counts and liver enzymes is mandatory in patients with pre-existing hepatic dysfunction.

Low-dose methotrexate (MTX)

Introduction of drug class

Methotrexate was introduced in the 1950s as a potent antifolate cytotoxic agent, primarily intended for chemotherapy. The drug is used extensively (off-label) in rheumatology. Tolerability limitations and pregnancy alerts make MTX the least favorable among the available immunomodulators.

Indications

Low-dose MTX may be recommended for induction of remission in steroid-refractory luminal Crohn's disease as well as for maintenance in Crohn's patients refractory or intolerant to thiopurines. Evidence of benefit in fistulizing Crohn's disease is limited, and there is no evidence to support the use of MTX in UC. The only prospective study available employed unusually low (12.5 mg/week) oral dosing and failed to show benefit. Two multicenter trials of parenteral MTX (METEOR and MERIT) are ongoing.

Co-administration with anti-TNF

The addition of subcutaneous MTX (25 mg weekly) to a loading dose of infliximab in Crohn's patients did not improve rates of steroid-free remission achieved by infliximab alone.

Basic pharmacology

Mechanism of action (Figure 7.2)

MTX is thought to affect cancer and inflammation by different mechanisms.

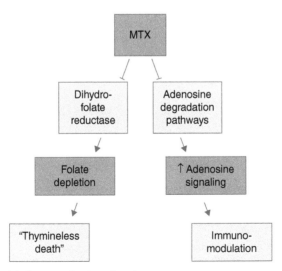

Figure 7.2 Mechanism of action of methotrexate.

Cytotoxic effect

In high doses, when used for the therapy of malignancies, MTX inhibits the enzyme dihydrofolate reductase, abrogating the conversion of dihydrofolate into active tetrahydrofolate. Tetrahydrofolate is essential for the synthesis of pyrimidine nucleotide thymidine. A decrease in thymidine in rapidly dividing tumor cells results in breakage of DNA replication forks, eventually triggering apoptosis, the phenomenon called "thymineless death."

Immunomodulatory effect

In low doses used in anti-inflammatory regimens, MTX mostly affects folate-dependent enzymes of purine metabolism, leading to the accumulation of adenosine. Adenosine exerts its immunoregulatory effect by acting on P1 adenosine receptors, preventing activation of T-cells and neutrophils.

Bioavailability

Absorption of MTX is dose-dependent and relatively unpredictable. Thus, parenteral administration should be preferred, at least for induction.

Metabolism

MTX enters cells by active transport and becomes trapped within the cell in form of polyglutamate compounds. Those long-live compounds explain protracted effect of the drug.

MTX does not undergo significant metabolism.

The main route of excretion is renal. Both glomerular filtration and tubular secretion play role in the excretion.

Main drug interaction (Table 7.5)

Caution should be exerted when co-administered with nephrotoxic agents, drugs that compete for tubular secretion, and concomitant myelotoxic agents.

Table 7.5 Main drug interactions

Drug	Interaction
Co-trimoxazole*	
Sulfonamide**	Compete for tubular clearance
Trimethoprim	Additive anti-folate effect
Penicillins	Compete for tubular clearance
Proton pump inhibitors	Compete for tubular clearance
NSAIDs	May reduce glomerular filtration*

*Undesirable combination.
**Sulfasalazine appears to be safe.

Adverse effects

Low-dose weekly regimens used for immunomodulation in IBD appear to be safe and relatively well tolerated.

Cytotoxic effect

Cytotoxic effects, including bone marrow suppression and hemorrhagic enteritis, are only rarely seen with low-dose weekly immunomodulatory regimens. If observed, cytotoxicity should immediately prompt an evaluation for erroneous (daily) dosing, impaired excretion (deterioration of renal function), and interfering drugs. Folinic acid (5-formyl derivative of tetrahydrofolic acid) bypasses the block in tetrahydrofolate production and can be used as an efficient rescue agent.

Gastrointestinal intolerability

Vague abdominal sypmptoms, mainly nausea and abdominal discomfort, are reported by up to 10% of patients; supplementation with folate may help in some.

Hepatotoxicity

Historical daily (psoriasis) oral regimens have been associated with significant liver toxicity. Improved (weekly) regimens, along with customary folate supplementation, significantly reduce this risk. Persistent elevation of liver transaminases warrants discontinuation of the treatment and further evaluation, including with liver biopsy.

Pulmonary toxicity

MTX-related interstitial pneumonitis is a rare, yet well described phenomenon.

The patient should be advised to seek medical attention if they develop dyspnea or a nonproductive cough. MTX-related pneumonitis usually responds to the cessation of MTX, yet may require corticosteroid therapy; progressive disease is uncommon.

Carcinogenicity

Chronic immunosuppression results in defective T-cell immunosurveillance, raising a concern for potential development of *lymphoproliferative disorders*.

Evidence is limited to case-reports of Epstein Barr virus-related non-Hodgkin lymphoma. A large retrospective arthritis study found no excessive risk of non-Hodgkin lymphoma.

Table 7.6 Pre-treatment evaluation

Induction	Complete blood count	Every 2-4 weeks
Maintenance	Liver transaminases	Every 2-3 months

Folate supplementation

This should be considered in all patients taking MTX. Once weekly 5 mg or 1 mg daily 5 days schedules are advised, but folate *should not* be taken on the same day as the MTX.

Pre-treatment evaluation

- Complete blood count (Table 7.6)
- Blood chemistry including BUN, creatinine and liver enzymes
- Hepatic sonography
- Chest X-ray.

Monitoring (Table 7.7)

Table 7.7 Monitoring

Finding	Action required
Myelosuppression • WBC < 3.5×10^9/L • PMN <2×10^9/L • Platelets <150×10^9/L	Withhold treatment Folinic acid rescue if severe
Macrocytosis	Start folate supplementation
Megaloblastic anemia	Withhold treatment Start folate supplementation
Oral ulceration, vomiting, diarrhea	Withhold treatment Rule out overdose (erroneous daily intake?) Start folate supplementation
ALT 2–3 times upper limits of normal (ULN)	Reduce dose
ALT > 3 times ULN	Withhold treatment Consider biopsy if persists
Deterioration of renal function	Discontinue immediately Nephrotoxic drugs?

Table 7.8 Adult dosing information			
Induction	25 mg Once Weekly	IM	Evaluate for response in 4–6 wks Continue for up to 16 wks
Maintenance	15 mg	IM, SC, PO	

Adult dosing information (Table 7.8)
Pediatric dosing information
Pediatric starting dose is 10–15 mg/m² once weekly.

Administration in hepatic or renal impairment
This is not recommended.

Pregnancy considerations
MTX is absolutely contraindicated (FDA X) for use during pregnancy. Teratogenic, abortofacient and spermotoxic effects are well described. Reliable contraception is mandatory for both females and males during MTX therapy and for six months following discontinuation.

In case of inadvertent pregnancy, patients should be advised to discontinue MTX immediately, discuss the situation with their obstetrician team, and consider the termination of pregnancy.

Breastfeeding
MTX is secreted into milk and is contraindicated for nursing patients.

Calcineurin inhibitors

- Approved for and widely used in transplant medicine.
- Intravenous (CsA) is a potent salvage therapy in acute severe steroid-refractory ulcerative colitis but has largely been replaced by infliximab for this indication.
- Tacrolimus may have some effect in Crohn's disease.

Basic pharmacology
Mechanism of action (Figure 7.3)
Clonal expansion of activated T-cells largely depends on autocrine IL2 signaling.

Engagement of the T-cell receptor results in activation of the calmodulin-calcineurin cascade. Activated calcineurin, in turn,

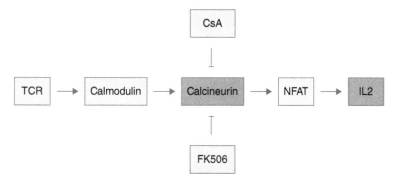

Figure 7.3 Mechanism of action of calcineurin inhibitors. CsA, cyclosporin A; FK506, tacrolimus; IL2, interleukin 2; NFAT, nuclear factor of activated T-cells; TCR, T-cell receptor.

dephosphorylates transcription factor NFAT, and subsequent nuclear translocation of NFAT initiates the production and release of IL2, leading to rapid proliferation of the activated cell. A small lipophylic peptide CsA and a macrolide tacrolimus (FK506) block the phosphorylase activity of calcineurin, effectively abrogating clonal expansion of the activated T-cells.

Bioavailability
Both drugs are only poorly (~ 20%) absorbed. If administered orally, CsA should be taken with a fatty meal; absorption of microemulsion formulation is less dependable on bile acids.

Metabolism
Both drugs are extensively metabolized by hepatic cytochrome P450 3A4 enzymes and excreted into the bile. Significant genetic polymorphism of P450 and abundant drug-induced variations in its activity result in great variability in blood levels of the medications. Blood level monitoring and level-based dose adjustment are thus obligatory.

Indications, dosing information and monitoring
Intravenous CsA is an effective "colon salvage therapy" in patients with severe steroid-refractory ulcerative colitis and in the past served as a "bridge" to maintenance therapy with the slowly acting thiopurines. Even a relatively short course of the treatment (one week) is frequently associated with significant and potentially life-threatening adverse events; presently, CsA has been largely replaced for biological agents (infliximab) for this indication.

On the "rescue" regimen, patients initially start on 2–4 mg/kg/day of CsA by continuous infusion; blood levels should be obtained starting from the second day of the treatment, and vigorously monitored (usually on an alternate day basis) with target of 150–250 ng/ml.

Blood pressure, renal function (both urinary output and serum creatinine and urea nitrogen), serum potassium and magnesium levels should be vigorously monitored. Hypomagnesemia is frequent and together with hypocholesterolemia (serum cholesterol less than 120 mg/dl) significantly increases the risk of seizures and should be avoided.

Responders are usually continued with oral CsA 8 mg/kg/day for an overlap period (2–3 months long) with thiopurines. Corticosteroids should be tapered during this overlap period. Prophylaxis against *Pneumocystis carinii* pneumonia for the entire triple immunosuppressive period is mandatory. If the patient relapses at any point, they should be referred for colectomy; second "rescue" with infliximab is associated significant risk of life-threatening opportunistic infection and should be avoided.

Adverse effects and toxicity

CsA and tacrolimus have similar safety profiles.

Major risks of rescue therapy with CsA are given in Table 7.9.

Risk of malignancy

Immunosuppression affects the ability of the immune system to recognize and to combat tumor cells. Long-term immunosuppression with calcineurin inhibitors (unusual in IBD regimens) is associated with an increased risk of skin cancer and lymphoproliferative disorders.

Table 7.9 Major risks of rescue therapy with CsA

Idiosyncrasy	Anaphylaxis 0.9%
Immunosuppression*	Severe infections (6.3%)
Vasospasm	Severe nephrotoxicity (5.4%)
	Hypertension (39%)
Neurotoxicity**	Seizures (3.6%)
	Paresthesias (51%)
Metabolic derangements	Hyperkalemia (13%)
	Hypomagnesemia (42%)
	Hyperglycemia

*Consider *Pneumocystis carinii* pneumonia (PCP) prophylaxis.
**Can be predicted by low serum cholesterol levels.

Table 7.10 Drug interactions

Increase CsA/tacrolimus levels	Decrease CsA/tacrolimus levels
Diltiazem, verapamil	
Ketoconazole, fluconazole	Phenobarbital, carbamazepine, phenytoin
Clarithromycin, erythromycin	Nafcillin, rifabutin, rifampin
Proton pump inhibitors	
Cimetidine	
Methylprednisolone	
Metaclopramide	Octreotide
Grapefruit juice	St. John's Wort

Drug interactions (Table 7.10)

A large variety of drugs can either induce or compete for hepatic P450 3A4 enzymes, significantly interfering with metabolism of calcineurin inhibitors. Periodic monitoring of drug levels is therefore the absolute necessity.

Pregnancy considerations (Category C)

Cyclosporine and tacrolimus lack genotoxic effects, yet may be associated with increased rates of prematurity. The drugs may be used during pregnancy when the potential benefits exceed the possible risk.

Breastfeeding

Both drugs appear in breast milk in substantial amounts and pose a risk of immunosuppression for the nursing infant; breastfeeding should thus be avoided.

Administration in patients with renal impairment

This should be avoided.

Recommended reading

Akbari M, Shah S, Velayos FS, *et al.* (2013) Systematic review and meta-analysis on the effects of thiopurines on birth outcomes from female and male patients with inflammatory bowel disease. *Inflamm Bowel Dis*; **19**: 15–22.

The most updated review of effects of thiopurines on pregnancy outcomes in inflammatory disease patients.

Thiopurine exposure in women with IBD was associated with preterm birth (OR 1.67, 95% CI 1.26 –2.20) but not with low birth weight (OR 1.01, 95% CI 0.96–1.06) or congenital abnormalities (OR 1.45, 95% CI 0.99–2.13).

Bastida G, Nos P, Aguas M, *et al.* (2005) Incidence, risk factors and clinical course of thiopurine-induced liver injury in patients with inflammatory bowel disease. *Aliment Pharmacol Ther* **22**: 775–82.

Beaugerie L, Brousse N, Bouvier AM, *et al.* (2009) Lymphoproliferative disorders in patients receiving thiopurines for inflammatory bowel disease: a prospective observational cohort study. *Lancet* **374**: 1617–25.
Landmark prospective nationwide French cohort study (by CESAME group) involving 19 486 IBD patients followed up for median 35 months (29–40) and addressing risk of lymphoproliferative complications associated with treatment with thiopurines. The incidence rates of lymphoproliferative disorder were:
On thiopurines (30.1%): 0.90/1000 patient-years
Past exposure (14.4%): 0.20/1000 patient-years
Never received thiopurines (55.5%): 0.26/1000 patient-years
Hazard ratio of lymphoproliferative disorder between patients receiving thiopurines and those who had never received the drugs was 5.28 (2.01–13.9, p=0.0007)

Ben-Horin S, Goldstein I, Fudim E, *et al.* (2009) Early preservation of effector functions followed by eventual T-cell memory depletion: a model for the delayed onset of the effect of thiopurines. *Gut* **58**: 396–403.

Chan ES, Cronstein BN (2010) Methotrexate: how does it really work? *Nat Rev Rheumatol* **6**: 175–8.
Important insight into mechanisms of anti-inflammatory activity of low-dose methotrexate.

Chande N, Abdelgadir I, Gregor J (2011) The safety and tolerability of methotrexate for treating patients with Crohn's disease. *J Clin Gastroenterol* **45**: 599–601.

Deepak P, Sifuentes H, Sherid M, *et al.* (2013) T-cell non-Hodgkin's lymphomas reported to the FDA AERS with tumor necrosis factor-alpha (TNF-alpha) inhibitors: results of the REFURBISH study. *Am J Gastroenterol* Jan.; **108**: 99–105.

Khan KJ, Dubinsky MC, Ford AC, et al. (2011) Efficacy of immunosuppressive therapy for inflammatory bowel disease: a systematic review and meta-analysis. *Am J Gastroenterol* **106**: 630–42.
Comprehensive systemic review addressing efficacy of immunomodulators in inflammatory bowel disease. There is no evidence to suggest the ability of AZA/6-MP to induce remission in either active Crohn's disease (5 RCTs, 380 patients) or ulcerative colitis (2 RCTs, 130 patients). In quiescent Crohn's disease, continuing thiopurines has been shown to successfully prevent relapse in 3 withdrawal trials. In quiescent UC, AZA has been shown to successfully maintain remission in 3 trials.

Kornbluth A, Sachar DB (2010) Ulcerative colitis practice guidelines in adults: American College Of Gastroenterology, Practice Parameters Committee. *Am J Gastroenterol* **105**: 501–23.

Lewis JD, Abramson O, Pascua M, *et al.* Timing of myelosuppression during thiopurine therapy for inflammatory bowel disease: implications for monitoring recommendations. *Clin Gastroenterol Hepatol* **7**: 1195–1201.

Lichtenstein GR, Hanauer SB, Sandborn WJ (2009) Management of Crohn's disease in adults. *Am J Gastroenterol* **104**: 465–83.

Lichtenstein GR, Feagan BG, Cohen RD, *et al.* (2012) Serious infection and mortality in patients with Crohn's disease: more than 5 years of follow-up in the TREAT registry. *Am J Gastroenterol* **107**: 1409–22.

Lichtiger S, Present DH, Kornbluth A, *et al.* (1994) Cyclosporine in severe ulcerative colitis refractory to steroid therapy. *N Engl J Med* **330**: 1841–5.
Landmark study addressing effect of cyclosporine on steroid-refractory acute severe ulcerative colitis; 9 of 11 (82%) steroid-refractory patients with acute severe ulcerative colitis were given a continuous infusion CsA dosed 4 mg/kg per day and responded within a mean of seven days; none of the 9 patients who were assigned to placebo improved spontaneously. Furthermore, all five patients initially treated with placebo, who were then given cyclosporine, also show a response.

McSharry K, Dalzell AM, Leiper K, *et al.* (2011) Systematic review: the role of tacrolimus in the management of Crohn's disease. *Aliment Pharmacol Ther* **34**: 1282–94.

Mayberry JF, Lobo A, Ford AC, *et al.* (2012) NICE clinical guideline (CG152): the management of Crohn's disease in adults, children and young people. *Aliment Pharmacol Ther* Nov.; **14**. Epub ahead of print.

Moder KG, Tefferi A, Cohen MD, *et al.* (1995) Hematologic malignancies and the use of methotrexate in rheumatoid arthritis: a retrospective study. *Am J Med* **99**: 276–81.

Mowat C, Cole A, Windsor A, *et al.* (2011) Guidelines for the management of inflammatory bowel disease in adults. *Gut* **60**: 571–607.

Oren R, Arber N, Odes S, *et al.* (1996) Methotrexate in chronic active ulcerative colitis: a double-blind, randomized, Israeli multicenter trial. *Gastroenterology* **110**: 1416–21.

Sparrow MP, Hande SA, Friedman S, *et al.* (2007) Effect of allopurinol on clinical outcomes in inflammatory bowel disease nonresponders to azathioprine or 6-mercaptopurine. *Clin Gastroenterol Hepatol* **5**: 209–14.

Sternthal MB, Murphy SJ, George J, *et al.* (2008) Adverse events associated with the use of cyclosporine in patients with inflammatory bowel disease. *Am J Gastroenterol* **103**: 937–43.

Van Assche G, Vermeire S, Rutgeerts P (2011) Management of acute severe ulcerative colitis. *Gut* **60**: 130–3.

Weinshilboum RM, Sladek SL (1980) Mercaptopurine pharmacogenetics: monogenic inheritance of erythrocyte thiopurine methyltransferase activity. *Am J Hum Genet* **32**: 651–62.
Landmark study addressing nuances of genetic variability of TPMT and their impact on metabolism of thiopurines. Erythrocyte (RBC) TPMT activity was measured in blood samples from 298 randomly selected subjects. Of the study subjects, high enzyme activity was demonstrated in 88.6% and intermediate activity in 11.1%; additional 0.3% of subjects had undetectable activity of TPMT.

CHAPTER 8

Biological agents
Gert Van Assche
Mount Sinai Hospital, Toronto, ON, Canada

Biological agents approved to treat IBD

All of the biological agents currently approved for the treatment of inflammatory bowel disease (IBD) are monoclonal antibodies (Table 8.1). Two antitumor necrosis factor (TNF) IgG1 antibodies, infliximab (Remicade®) and adalimumab (Hunira®), and one pegylated Fab antibody fragment, certolizumab-pegol (Cimzia®), have demonstrated efficacy in the treatment of refractory luminal Crohn's disease (CD). Infliximab is a chimeric mouse-human antibody, certolizumab is a humanized Fab fragment. Golimumab (Simponi®) and adalimumab are fully human antibodies. The human TNF receptor-Fc fragment construct, etanercept (Enbrel®), has failed to show efficacy in Crohn's disease. The pleotropic inflammatory cytokine, TNF, is secreted by several immune cells, predominantly by monocytes and, after binding to one of its 2 receptors, induces several pro-inflammatory signals in immune and nonimmune cells. Inhibition of TNF signalling results in apoptosis of activated T-cells, decreased cytokine secretion, reduction of leukocyte migration and restoration of the mucosal barrier of the gut. Only infliximab is approved by the European and American authorities to treat perianal fistulizing CD. Also, scheduled maintenance therapy with infliximab and adalimumab results in more pronounced mucosal healing and is associated with a reduction in disease-related hospitalizations. In ulcerative colitis (UC), infliximab, adalimumab and golimumab induce and maintain remission and result in mucosal healing in treatment-refractory moderate-to-severe disease. In addition, infliximab is efficacious in decreasing the risk of colectomy in steroid refractory hospitalized patients with severe attacks of UC.

Infliximab is administered intravenously at a dose of 5 mg/kg at week 0, 2 and 6 for induction and afterwards every 8 weeks as maintenance therapy. Adalimumab induction therapy consists of two doses given subcutaneously (SC) 2 weeks apart. Depending on disease severity, 80/40 mg or 160/80 mg is used at induction. Maintenance therapy consists of 40 mg

Pocket Guide to Gastrointestinal Drugs, Edited by M. Michael Wolfe and Robert C. Lowe. © 2014 John Wiley & Sons, Ltd. Published 2014 by John Wiley & Sons, Ltd.

Table 8.1 Biological agents approved for IBD with their respective recommended dosing

Generic name	Trade name	Indication	Approved in	Dosing schedule
Anti-TNF agents				
Infliximab	Remicade	CD, UC	Worldwide	5 mg/kg IV 0,2,6 wks and q8 wks IV maintenance
Adalimumab	Humira	CD, UC	Worldwide for CD EU and USA for UC	160/80 mg or 80/40 SC induction and q2 wks 40 mg SC maintenance
Golimumab	Simponi	UC	USA	200/100 mg SC induction and q4 wks 100 mg SC maintenance
Certolizumab-pegol	Cimzia	CD	USA, Switzerland	400 mg SC wk 0,2 4 and q4 wks maintenance
Anti-integrins				
Natalizumab	Tysabri	CD	USA	300 mg IV q4 wks maintenance

CD, Crohn's disease; EU, European Union, UC, ulcerative colitis, USA, United States of America.

administered every 2 weeks. Golimumab has been approved by the FDA in May 2013 for the induction and maintenance of ulcerative colitis at a dose of 200 mg SC, followed by 100 mg SC after 2 weeks and 100 mg maintenance every 4 weeks thereafter. Approval in other jurisdictions around the world is pending.

For children and adolescents with IBD, anti-TNF antibodies have become available more recently. Currently, infliximab and adalimumab are approved in the USA, Canada and in Europe for pediatric CD and infliximab for pediatric UC. Dosing per kilogram is identical to that used in adults. Since adalimumab dosing is not weight-based, the induction and maintenance doses are adapted for children who are underweight. Certolizumab-pegol has not been studied for pediatric IBD.

Natalizumab (Tysabri®), an anti-α_4 integrin IgG4 antibody and the first representative of a new class of biological agents, the anti-adhesion molecules, maintains steroid free clinical remission in luminal Crohn's disease. The drug is efficacious in patients failing anti-TNF therapy. However, due to the risk of progressive multifocal encephalopathy (PML), a potentially lethal brain infection caused by JC virus reactivation, the FDA has approved its use only for patients failing anti-TNF therapy and in a tight pharmacovigilance program. The antibody has not been approved by Health Canada or by the European Medicines Agency (EMA). Several, more gut-selective, anti-adhesion molecules are in clinical development and clinical efficacy has been shown in ulcerative colitis for the IgG2 monoclonal antibody, vedolizumab.

Optimal treatment strategies with anti TNF therapies in IBD

Infliximab had been used episodically, in an on-flare treatment strategy, in the early years after it became initially available. However, interrupted use with long drug holidays results more often in the formation of antidrug antibodies associated with severe infusion reactions and with loss of response. In addition, repeated flares of Crohn's disease most likely lead to cumulative intestinal damage and increase the risk of surgery and subsequent loss of organ function. Therefore, induction followed by scheduled maintenance therapy has become the standard of care for anti-TNF therapies in IBD. Whether anti-TNF therapies should be started as early as possible after diagnosis is more controversial. In Crohn's disease, retrospective cohort studies indicate that young patients and those with perianal disease or extensive small bowel disease are at an increased risk of a rapidly progressing disease course. Those patients are prime candidates for early intervention with biological agents. Also, patients who present with a severe attack of UC and fail to respond to a short course of IV steroids, should be considered for medical rescue therapy with infliximab. Conversely, reliable predictors of a benign disease course are currently not available in UC and in CD. Evidence from a prospectively recruited cohort in Southern Norway suggests that symptom control can be obtained without biological agents in 43% of patients with CD and 55% of those with UC after the initial flare, but it is unclear if long-term organ damage is also prevented in this population.

Another important isue is the concomitant administration of immunosuppressive therapy with anti-TNF agents. In rheumatoid arthritis, methotrexate combined with infliximab and adalimumab has consistently been shown to increase therapeutic efficacy. In Crohn's disease, the best evidence to support the use of combination therapy at the start of anti-TNF therapy comes from the blinded double-dummy controlled SONIC trial comparing azathioprine monotherapy (2.5 mg/kg/d), infliximab monotherapy (5 mg/kg IV at wk 0, 2 and 6 and every 8 weeks until one year) and combined infliximab plus azathioprine therapy. At 26 weeks the steroid free remission rates in patients receiving combined immunosuppressive therapy with infliximab and azathioprine were higher than with infliximab or azathioprine monotherapy. In contrast, it has not been conclusively established how long the combination of both biological and immunosuppressive agents needs to be continued. Withdrawal of azathioprine from patients in durable clinical remission on combination therapy has been tested in one controlled trial with a limited number of patients and withdrawal of infliximab has been tested in one uncontrolled prospective cohort study. Prospective data on the therapeutic benefit of combining immunosuppressives such as azathioprine with adalimumab, golimumab or certolizumab pegol are lacking.

Safety of biological agents in IBD

Anti-TNF therapies act by dampening the response of the human immune system to inflammatory triggers and therefore increase the risk of serious infections. Infections with intracellular pathogens such as mycobacteria and histoplasma have been a specific concern and warnings regarding both of these diseases have been included in the package inserts. Other serious infections, including CD-associated abdominal or perianal sepsis, are also more prevalent in patients treated with biological agents and both patients and physicians should be aware of these risks. The overall risk of malignancy is not increased in patients with IBD treated with biologicals although some specific neoplasms have been associated with combined use of anti-TNF agents and azathioprine. Non-Hodgkin lymphomas, including hepatosplenic T-cell lymphomas, are more prevalent in patients on anti-TNF therapy although the absolute risk is very low and the relative contribution of azathioprine to this elevated risk needs to be studied further. Specific risks associated with anti-TNF agents include the progression of advanced congestive heart failure and the worsening of demyelinating neurologic disease. Autoimmune disease associated with the presence of antinuclear, notably of anti-ds-DNA antibodies, is a rare complication of chronic anti TNF therapy and symptoms vary from eczematous skin lesions to drug-induced lupus. The risk of PML, a serious brain infection, in patients treated with natalizumab, has been discussed earlier.

Most anti-TNF agents approved for use in IBD are FDA Pregnancy Category B with the exception of natalizumab, which is category C.

Emerging biologicals

Novel biologicals are being developed for the treatment of patients failing standard therapies including the available anti-TNF antibodies. For ulcerative colitis, inhibition of gut selective integrins with vedolizumab has shown preliminary efficacy in both UC and CD. Other selective anti-adhesion molecules are being developed and this class of agent may offer an improved benefit-to-risk profile due to the lack of systemic immunosuppression. These drugs are the first class of agents that are specifically developed for gastrointestinal disease, as they are not expected to be efficacious for nongastrointestinal disorders. Ustekinumab, an anti-IL12/23 p40 antibody, has also shown efficacy in Crohn's disease, particularly in previous anti-TNF failures.

Recommended reading

Baert F, Noman M, Vermeire S, *et al*. (2003) Influence of immunogenicity on the long-term efficacy of infliximab in Crohn's disease. *N Engl J Med* **348**: 601–8.

Behm BW, Bickston SJ (2008) Tumor necrosis factor-alpha antibody for maintenance of remission in Crohn's disease. *Cochrane Database Syst Rev*: CD006893.
Systematic meta-analysis of all clinical trials with anti-TNF agents in Crohn's disease and conclude that at least for maintenance therapy all agents are equivalent.

Colombel JF, Sandborn WJ, Reinisch W, *et al*. (2010) Infliximab, azathioprine, or combination therapy for Crohn's disease. *N Engl J Med* Apr.; **362**(15): 1383–95. PubMed PMID: 20393175.

D'Haens G, Baert F, van Assche G, Caenepeel P, *et al*. (2008) Early combined immunosuppression or conventional management in patients with newly diagnosed Crohn's disease: an open randomised trial. *Lancet* **371**: 660–7.

Hanauer SB, Feagan BG, Lichtenstein GR, *et al*. (2002) Maintenance infliximab for Crohn's disease: the ACCENT I randomised trial. *Lancet* **359**: 1541–9.

Hanauer SB, Sandborn WJ, Rutgeerts P, *et al*. (2006) Human anti-tumor necrosis factor monoclonal antibody (adalimumab) in Crohn's disease: the CLASSIC-I trial. *Gastroenterology* Feb.; **130**(2): 323–33.

Laharie D, Bourreille A, Branche J, *et al*. (2012) Ciclosporin versus infliximab in patients with severe ulcerative colitis refractory to intravenous steroids: a parallel, open-label randomised controlled trial. *Lancet* Dec.; **380**(9857): 1909–15.

Louis E, Mary JY, Vernier-Massouille G, *et al*. (2012) Maintenance of remission among patients with Crohn's disease on antimetabolite therapy after infliximab therapy is stopped. *Gastroenterology* **142**: 63–70.
Prospective cohort study investigating the impact of withdrawing infliximab in patients with Crohn's disease in durable remission with a combination of infliximab and azathioprine.

Rutgeerts P, Sandborn WJ, Feagan BG, *et al*. (2005) Infliximab for induction and maintenance therapy for ulcerative colitis. *N Engl J Med* **353**: 2462.

Rutgeerts P, Van Assche G, Sandborn WJ, *et al*. (2012) Adalimumab induces and maintains mucosal healing in patients with Crohn's disease: Data from the

EXTEND Trial. *Gastroenterology* Feb 8. [Epub ahead of print] PubMed PMID: 22326435.

Sandborn WJ, Colombel JF, Enns R *et al.* (2005) Natalizumab induction and maintenance therapy for Crohn's disease. *N Engl J Med* **353**: 1912–25.

Sandborn WJ, Feagan BG, Stoinov S, *et al.* (2007) Certolizumab pegol for the treatment of Crohn's disease. *N Engl J Med* **357**: 228–38.

Sandborn WJ, van Assche G, Reinisch W, *et al.* (2012a) Adalimumab induces and maintains clinical remission in patients with moderate-to-severe ulcerative colitis. *Gastroenterology* Feb.; **142**(2): 257–65.

Sandborn WJ, Gasink C, Gao LL, *et al.* (2012b) Ustekinumab induction and maintenance therapy in refractory Crohn's disease. *N Engl J Med* **367**: 1519–28.
Randomized trial demonstrating the efficacy of ustekinumab in Crohn's disease. Notably patients resistant to infliximab showed an enhanced response.

Schreiber S, Khaliq-Kareemi M, Lawrance IC *et al.* (2007) Maintenance therapy with certolizumab pegol for Crohn's disease. *N Engl J Med* **357**: 239–50.

Targan SR, Feagan BG, Fedorak RN *et al.* (2007) Natalizumab for the treatment of active Crohn's disease: results of the ENCORE Trial. *Gastroenterology* May; **132**: 1672–83.
Randomized trial with the anti-integrin Ab natalizulab, which demonstrates its clinical activity, particularly in maintenance, in patients failing infliximab therapy.

Van Assche G, Magdelaine-Beuzelin C, D'Haens G, *et al.* (2008) Withdrawal of immunosuppression in Crohn's disease treated with scheduled infliximab maintenance: a randomized trial. *Gastroenterology* **134**: 1861–8.
Randomized study in patients on long term combined anti TNF therapy and immunosuppressive therapy. The data indicate that withdrawal of immunosuppressives after 6 months does not affect clinical outcomes with continued infliximab therapy.

Van Assche G, Lewis JD, Lichtenstein GR, *et al.* (2011) The London position statement of the World Congress of Gastroenterology on Biological Therapy for IBD with the European Crohn's and Colitis Organisation: safety. *Am J Gastroenterol* Sep.; **106**(9): 1594–1602.

LIVER AND PANCREAS

PART III

CHAPTER 9

Interferons

Robert C. Lowe
Boston University School of Medicine, Boston, MA, USA

Introduction

Interferons were first described by Isaacs and Lindenmann in 1957 as a group of unknown factors that "interfered" with the replication of influenza virus in an experimental chicken egg model. The molecules themselves were isolated in the 1970s, and they are currently identified as a superfamily of more than 20 proteins with diverse roles in the immune response to exogenous pathogens. They are utilized clinically in the treatment of viral infections, neurological disorders, congenital immune deficiency diseases, and as a component of chemotherapy regimens for a select group of malignancies.

Mechanism of action

Interferons are produced as part of the innate immune response when pathogen-associated molecular patterns (PAMPs) are recognized by Toll-like receptors and other recognition molecules on the surface and within the cytoplasm of dendritic cells. Interferons alpha, beta, and gamma have roles in innate immunity, but only IFN alpha has been used in the therapy of gastrointestinal disorders, specifically viral hepatitis B and C. Interferon beta has been proven effective in the treatment of multiple sclerosis, while IFN gamma has a role in the therapy of two rare conditions – chronic granulomatous disease and osteopetrosis. Interferon lambda is currently being studied in the treatment of chronic hepatitis C infection, but these studies are preliminary and there are currently no approved formulations for this indication. Interferon alpha is also a component of therapy for selected malignancies, including renal cell cancer, melanoma, hairy cell leukemia, lymphoma, multiple myeloma, and AIDS-related Kaposi's sarcoma.

Interferon alpha acts by binding to a cell surface receptor (IFNAR), inducing a signaling cascade involving the JAK-STAT pathway, leading

Pocket Guide to Gastrointestinal Drugs, Edited by M. Michael Wolfe and Robert C. Lowe. © 2014 John Wiley & Sons, Ltd. Published 2014 by John Wiley & Sons, Ltd.

to the translocation of transcription factors to the cell nucleus and subsequent transcription of a number of cytokines and other proteins that both directly inhibit viral replication and stimulate helper T-cells to promote immune-mediated destruction of virus-infected hepatocytes. Interferons alpha and beta bind the same set of cell surface receptors, which are present on a wide variety of cell types. In contrast, interferon lambda binds a different set of receptors with a more restricted distribution, being expressed on primarily on hepatocytes but not on vascular endothelium or cells of the CNS; this limited distribution gives interferon lambda a much better side effect profile than interferon alpha, stimulating research into its use as therapy in chronic hepatitis

Pharmacology

IFN alpha is a polypeptide comprised of more than 160 amino acids, and thus is not orally bioavailable. Standard IFN alpha is administered by subcutaneous injection, with rapid absorption (peak levels occur within 12 hours) and rapid elimination via renal clearance. As such, therapy with IFN requires thrice-weekly injections, and serum drug levels fluctuate greatly throughout the week. Viral kinetic studies demonstrate that during the IFN trough, hepatitis C virus (HCV) levels rise, leading to a cycling of viral loads that contributes to the low rate of efficacy of this early HCV treatment; studies demonstrated only a 10–20% rate of sustained viral response after 48 weeks of therapy.

A major advance in IFN-based therapy came in 2001 with the development and testing of pegylated interferon molecules. These drugs consist of an interferon alpha polypeptide complexed to a large polyethylene glycol (PEG) molecule. The addition of PEG slows the renal clearance of interferon, decreases the volume of distribution of the drug, and promotes a slow and sustained absorption of IFN, leading to maintenance of high serum drug levels for several days after a single subcutaneous injection. The presence of the large carbohydrate molecule, however, creates steric interference at the interferon receptor, making each molecule less effective at binding to and activating the receptor; thus there is a tradeoff between serum drug level and per-molecule efficacy.

There are two commonly used formulations of pegylated interferon, which differ in their structure and pharmacologic properties. PEG-IFN alpha 2a (Pegasys$_{TM}$) has a large PEG molecule (40 kDa) complexed to IFN by an amide bond at a lysine residue. This strong covalent bond is responsible for the long serum half-life of this formulation (approximately 65 hrs), and its slow clearance not by the kidney, but by nonspecific serum protease activity. On the other hand, the large PEG molecule significantly limits the activity of the interferon component, resulting in < 10% of the antiviral activity of the noncomplexed molecule. The other commonly used pegylated interferon molecule is PEG-IFN alpha 2b (PEG-Intron$_{TM}$), in which the IFN moiety is bound to a smaller (12 kDa) PEG molecule via a weaker bond at a histidine residue. This allows dissociation of the PEG from the IFN in about 50% of each dose, resulting in a longer serum half-life than standard interferon (approximately 30 hours), but not as prolonged as that of PEG-IFN alpha 2a. The efficacy of PEG-IFN alpha 2b, however, is nearly 30% that of the uncomplexed molecule due to the lesser degree of steric hindrance at the IFN receptor. The smaller PEG molecule also leads to an increased volume of distribution of drug, and as a result this formulation is dosed according to body weight, unlike the fixed dosing of PEG-IFN alpha 2a. It is clear that the two PEG-IFN molecules make different tradeoffs between per-molecule effectiveness and improved pharmacokinetics.

A recombinant form of alpha interferon was developed in 1996; this molecule, known as Interferon Alphacon-1 (Infergen$_{TM}$), is designed to mimic the most common amino acid sequences from the known forms of alpha interferon, and is thus deemed a "consensus interferon." It requires daily subcutaneous injection when used in combination with ribavirin for HCV treatment, and has thus not been widely used in the era of pegylated interferon therapies.

Clinical effectiveness

The major interferon used in gastroenterological therapeutics is alpha interferon, which in 1986 was discovered to be effective in the treatment of chronic hepatitis C infection. Single agent interferon, given subcutaneously at a dose of 6 million units three times per week, was approximately 10–20% effective in sustained viral eradication. This poor response rate limited the utility of this formulation, especially given the extensive side effect profile of interferons (see below). A major advance in HCV therapy came in the early years of the twenty-first century, when several studies demonstrated that the use of pegylated interferon in combination with the oral antiviral dug ribavirin increased the rate of sustained viral response (SVR) to 40% in genotype I HCV infection and 75-80% in genotype 2 and 3 infection. The two regimens available for chronic HCV treatment consisted of PEG-IFN alpha 2a at a dose of 180 mcg administered subcutaneously once per week along with weight-based oral ribavirin, versus weekly PEG-IFN alpha 2b at a dose of 1.5 mcg/kg along with weight-based oral ribavirin. Dose reductions were specified if neutropenia or severe thrombocytopenia were to occur. Comparison of these two regimens in retrospective studies produced conflicting results, but two randomized controlled prospective trials published in 2009–2010 reported improved SVR rates in the regimens containing PEG-IFN alpha 2a, while a third randomized controlled trial reported similar efficacy of the two PEG-IFN formulations; this trial, however, has been criticized for differences in ribavirin dosing that may have led to more relapses in the PEG-IFN alpha 2a group.

Dual therapy with pegylated IFN and ribavirin had been the mainstay of HCV therapy until 2011, when new direct-acting antiviral medications (DAAs) became available. Telaprevir and boceprevir, inhibitors of HCV viral protease activity, were the first DAAs to be approved for use by the FDA, The addition of telaprevir or boceprevir to regimens containing pegylated interferon and ribavirin improves SVR to 60–75% for patients with genotype 1 HCV, and "triple therapy" regimens are now the standard of care in the treatment of genotype 1 HCV infection. Patients with Genotype 2 and 3 HCV infection continue to be treated with dual therapy, as the addition of DAAs does not appear to improve rates of viral eradication for these genotypes.

Toxicity

Interferons are well known to cause numerous adverse effects. The most common of these are fatigue, fevers, chills, and arthralgias, mimicking the systemic response to an acute viral infection. These symptoms are reported to occur in 25–60% of patients using pegylated interferon for the treatment of chronic hepatitis C, and tend to be worst in the 1–2 days following the weekly subcutaneous injection. Patients may also experience irritability and difficulty with concentration or memory. Depression, which occurred in 20–30% of patients in the pivotal trials of HCV therapy, is a major concern for patients taking interferon, as suicidality has been reported. Treatment with SSRIs or other antidepressants is effective in ameliorating the depressive effects of interferon. More rarely, psychotic episodes have occurred in patients on interferon therapy, especially in those with a known history of bipolar disorder or other thought disorders; these psychotic episodes respond to standard antipsychotic therapy and remit after discontinuation of interferon. Other side effects include acute thyroiditis, which can be reversible, and the exacerbation of pre-existing autoimmune conditions such as SLE, sarcoidosis, and rheumatoid arthritis.

Interferons also have myelosuppressive effects, and both neutropenia and thrombocytopenia are commonly reported. Thus, patients taking interferon for the treatment of HCV are required to have neutrophil and platelet monitoring once per month. More rarely, acute pneumonitis manifesting as cough and dyspnea, has been reported, which may require prolonged therapy with corticosteroids. The two commonly used formulations of PEG-IFN have similar side effect profiles, though PEG-IFN alpha 2a has a more potent myelosuppressive effect than PEG-IFN alpha 2b.

All interferons are pregnancy category C, but it should be noted that all the currently approved regimens for HCV therapy include the use of ribavirin, which is highly teratogenic (pregnancy category X). For this reason, patients on HCV therapy must make every effort to prevent pregnancy, and two forms of birth control are recommended for the duration of therapy and for six months following treatment (to permit complete washout of ribavirin).

Interferon types with generic and brand names

See Table 9.1.

Table 9.1 Interferon types with generic and brand names

Generic	Brand Name
Interferon alfa-2a:	Roferon-A
Interferon alfa-2b:	Intron-A
PEGinterferon alfa-2a:	Pegasys
PEGinterferon alfa-2b:	Pegintron
Interferon alfa-n3:	Alferon-N
Interferon alfacon 1:	Infergen
Interferon beta-1a:	Avonex, Rebif
Interferon beta-1b:	Betaseron, Extavia
Interferon gamma-1b:	Actimmune
Interferon lambda – investigational, not available for use	

Table 9.2 Pregnancy classes

Generic	Brand Name	Class
Interferon alfa-2a:	Roferon-A	C
Interferon alfa-2b:	Intron-A	C
PEGinterferon alfa-2a:	Pegasys	C
PEGinterferon alfa-2b:	Pegintron	C
Interferon alfa-n3:	Alferon-N	C
Interferon alfacon 1:	Infergen	C
Interferon beta-1a:	Avonex, Rebif	C
Interferon beta-1b:	Betaseron, Extavia	C
Interferon gamma-1b:	Actimmune	C

Pregnancy classes

See Table 9.2.

Category C

Animal reproduction studies have shown an adverse effect on the fetus and there are no adequate and well-controlled studies in humans, but potential benefits may warrant use of the drug in pregnant women despite potential risks.

Initial interferon dosing regimens for chronic hepatitis C

- Interferon alpha: 3 million units sc three times per week
- Pegylated interferon alpha 2a: 180 mcg sc weekly
- Pegylated interferon alpha 2b: 1.5 mcg/kg sc weekly
- Interferon alfacon 1: 15 mcg sc daily

These doses may be modified if patients develop neutropenia or severe thrombocytopenia.

Duration of therapy is 24–48 weeks, determined by the adjunctive therapy being used (ribavirin ± DAA), HCV genotype, presence of cirrhosis, and response to previous IFN-based therapies. sc = subcutaneous injection.

Recommended reading

Aghemo A, Rumi MG, Colombo M (2010) Pegylated interferons alpha 2a and alpha 2b in the treatment of chronic hepatitis C. *Nat Rev Gastroenterol Hepatol* **7**: 485–94.

Ascione A, De Luca M, Tartaglione MT, *et al.* (2010) Peginterferon alfa-2a plus ribavirin is more effective than peginterferon alfa-2b plus ribavirin for treating chronic hepatitis C virus infection. *Gastroenterology* **138**: 116–22.
This study compared regimens containing PEG-IFN alpha 2a and 2b with equivalent ribavirin dosing, and demonstrated significantly higher SVR rates in the PEG-IFN alpha 2a group (68.8% vs 54.4%).

Bacon BR, Gordon SC, Lawitz E, *et al.* (2011) Boceprevir for previously treated chronic HCV genotype 1 infection. *N Engl J Med* **364**: 1207–17.

Bruno R, Sacci P, Cima S, *et al.* (2012) Comparison of Peinterferon pharmacokinetic and pharmacodynamic profiles. *J Viral Hepatitis* **19**: 33–6.
Excellent review comparing the pharmacodynamic and pharmacokinetic properties of PEG-interferon alpha 2a and 2b, outlining the differences in structure, drug absorption, clearance, and per-molecule efficacy between these formulations.

Fried MW, Shiffman ML, Reddy KR, *et al.* (2002) Peginterferon alfa-2a plus ribavirin for chronic hepatitis C virus infection. *N Engl J Med* **347**: 975–82.

George PM, Badiger R, Alazawi W, *et al.* (2012) Pharmacology and therapeutic potential of interferons. *Pharmacol and Therapeutics* **135**: 44–53.

Hadziyannis SJ, Sette H Jr, Morgan TR, *et al.* (2004) Peginterferon-alpha2a and ribavirin combination therapy in chronic hepatitis C: a randomized study of treatment duration and ribavirin dose. *Ann Intern Med* **140**: 346–55.

Hezode C, Forestier N, Dusheiko G, *et al.* (2009) Telaprevir and peginterferon with or without ribavirin for chronic HCV infection. *N Engl J Med* **360**: 1839–50.

Hoofnagle JH, Mullen KD, Jones DB, *et al.* (1986) Treatment of chronic non-A, non-B hepatitis with recombinant human alpha interferon: a preliminary report. *NEJM* **315**: 1575–8.
The first report of interferon as a therapy for chronic Hepatitis C (known at the time as non-A, non-B hepatitis), in which 10 patients received interferon monotherapy. Transaminase levels improved significantly in 80% of treated patients, and liver histology was also shown to improve.

Kwo PY, Lawitz EJ, McCone J, *et al.* (2010) Efficacy of boceprevir, an NS3 protease inhibitor, in combination with peginterferon alfa-2b and ribavirin in treatment-naive patients with genotype 1 hepatitis C infection (SPRINT-1): an open-label, randomised, multicentre phase 2 trial. *Lancet* **376**: 705–16.

Manns MP, McHutchison JG, Gordon SC, *et al.* (2001) Peginterferon alfa-2b plus ribavirin compared with interferon alfa-2b plus ribavirin for initial treatment of chronic hepatitis C: a randomised trial. *Lancet* **358**: 958–65.

McHutchison JG, Lawitz EJ, Shiffman ML, *et al.* (2009) Peginterferon alfa-2b or alfa-2a with ribavirin for treatment of hepatitis C infection. *N Engl J Med* **361**: 580–93.
This trial, known as the IDEAL study, compared PEG-IFN alpha 2a and 2b regimens, and reported similar SVR rates, but the high rate of viral relapse in the PEG-IFN alpha 2a cohort was much higher than in previous trials or subsequent studies that reported

better SVR efficacy for PEG-IFN alpha 2a-containing regimens. This anomalous relapse rate may be explained by differences in ribavirin dosing in the two arms of the IDEAL study, which were not present in later trials.

McHutchison JG, Everson GT, Gordon SC, *et al.* (2009) Telaprevir with peginterferon and ribavirin for chronic HCV genotype 1 infection. *N Engl J Med* **360**: 1827–38.

A pivotal trial of the DAA telaprevir with PEG-IFN and ribavirin for the treatment of chronic HCV infection, demonstrating an SVR of 61% for patients receiving 12 weeks of telaprevir with 24 weeks of PEG-IFN alpha 2a and ribavirin.

Poordad F, McCone J Jr, Bacon BR, *et al.* (2011) Boceprevir for untreated chronic HCV genotype 1 infection. *N Engl J Med* **364**: 1195–1206.

A pivotal trial of the DAA boceprevir with PEG-IFN and ribavirin for the treatment of chronic HCV infection, demonstrating an SVR of 67% for patients receiving boceprevir with PEG-IFN alpha 2a and ribavirin.

Rumi MG, Aghemo A, Prati GM, *et al.* (2010) Randomized study of peginterferon-alpha2a plus ribavirin vs peginterferon-alpha2b plus ribavirin in chronic hepatitis C. *Gastroenterology* **138**: 108–15.

This study compared regimens containing PEG-IFN alpha 2a and 2b with equivalent ribavirin dosing, and demonstrated significantly higher SVR rates in the alpha 2a group (66% vs 54%).

CHAPTER 10

Nucleoside analogs

Uri Avissar[1] and David P. Nunes[2]

[1]Boston University School of Medicine, Boston, MA, USA
[2]Boston University School of Medicine, Boston, MA, USA

Introduction

The introduction and approval of acyclovir in 1982 heralded an era of oral antiviral medications that have been used to treat herpesviruses (HSV 1 and 2, VZV), hepadnaviruses (hepatitis B), flaviviruses (hepatitis C), and lentiviruses (HIV), among others. Acyclovir, an acyclic guanine nucleoside analog (NA), is also a prototype of the nucleos(t)ide class of oral antivirals which act by inhibition of viral polymerase or reverse transcriptase. These nucleos(t)ide reverse transcriptase inhibitors (NRTI), some of which were initially used for treatment of HIV, have been found to be effective against hepatitis B. The nucleos(t)ide analogs (NAs) used for the treatment of hepatitis B fall into three structural categories: L-nucleoside analogs (lamivudine, telbivudine and emtricitabine), acyclic phosphonates (adefovir and tenofovir), and cyclopentane rings (entecavir).

The first antiviral agents used for the treatment of hepatitis B were the interferons (see above, Chapter 9). Their use has been limited by their side effects and limited efficacy. However, they have the advantage of a defined course of treatment, absence of viral resistance, and a broad antiviral activity. Furthermore rates of hepatitis B e and surface antigen seroconversion are higher than those achieved with nucleos(t)ide analogs used over a similar duration. Nucleos(t)ide analogs offer a more favorable adverse event profile, oral administration, and unlike interferons, can in most instances be used safely in patients with advanced liver disease. They carry the disadvantages of resistance development and need for long-term viral suppression.

Lamivudine, an L-nucleoside analog, became the first oral medication approved for chronic hepatitis B (CHB) in 1998. While very well tolerated it is no longer a first-line agent because long-term use results in high rates of viral resistance. Adefovir, an acyclic nucleotide analog,

Pocket Guide to Gastrointestinal Drugs, Edited by M. Michael Wolfe and Robert C. Lowe. © 2014 John Wiley & Sons, Ltd. Published 2014 by John Wiley & Sons, Ltd.

Table 10.1 Nucleos(t)ides used in hepatitis B and C

Generic name	Lamivudine	Telbivudine	Entecavir	Adefovir	Tenofovir	Ribavirin
Brand name	Epivir HBV	Tyzeka	Baraclude	Hepsera	Viread	Copegus, Rebetol
Structural Class	L-Nucleoside Analog		Cyclopentane ring	Acyclic phosphate		D-ribose sugar
Heterocyclic base	Cytidine	Thymidine	Guanosine	Adenosine	Adenosine	Triazole carboxamide (*guanosine*)
Pregnancy risk factor	C	B	C	C	B	X
Lactation	CI$^{¥}$	CI$^{¥}$	CI$^{¥}$	CI$^{¥}$	CI$^{¥}$	CI$^{¥}$
Tablet dose (mg/tab)	100 mg/tab	600 mg/tab	0.5 or 1 mg/tab	10 mg/tab	300 mg/tab	200 mg/tab
Daily dosing * regimen (mg/day)	100 mg (one tab)/day	600 mg (one tab)/day	NA naïve: 0.5 mg LMVr: 1mg†	10 mg/day	300 mg/day	Algorithm specific‡

*Dose requires renal adjustment.

$^{¥}$CI = contraindicated; insufficient data.

†NA= nucleoside analogue; use the 1mg dose in LMVr (lamivudine resistant virus) and in cirrhotic patients.

‡Total daily dose (given in two divided doses) for combination HCV treatment varies by genotype and patient weight. In general, Genotype 1 and 4: patient weight <75kg =1000 mg; patient weight >75 kg =1200 mg; genotype 2 and 3: 800 mg.

which was also first developed for the treatment of HIV, was approved at a lower dose for the treatment of hepatitis B in 2002. Unfortunately, it too suffered from high resistance rates and a risk of kidney toxicity with long-term use. In 2005, entecavir, a guanosine nucleoside analog, was introduced and has demonstrated excellent long-term efficacy with low rates of viral resistance. This was followed in 2008 by the approval of tenofovir, an acyclic phosphonate diester of adenosine monophosphate, which had also been developed for the treatment of HIV and was found to be a potent inhibitor or HBV DNA polymerase. Like entecavir, it is associated with low levels of viral resistance even with long-term use. Both now serve as first-line therapy for CHB. Other nucleoside analogs with activity against hepatitis B include the L-thymidine analog telbivudine and emtricitabine, a cytidine analog similar to lamivudine (Table 10.1).

Combination treatments with interferon and a NA have not been shown to increase efficacy in the treatment of CHB but this is an area which continues to be investigated. However, combination of ribavirin, a guanosine nucleoside analog, with interferon and a protease inhibitor, has become the cornerstone of chronic hepatitis C treatment. The mechanism of action of ribavirin is incompletely understood and is likely multifaceted. It is hence described separately in this chapter.

Mechanism of action

The nucleos(t)ide analogs enter cells by passive diffusion and possibly a carrier-mediated process. Nucleos(t)ide analogs require phosphorylation by either host cytoplasmic or viral kinases to form the active triphosphate substrate. While the L-nucleoside analogs and cyclopentane rings (a nucleoside analog) require three phosphorylations, the acyclic phosphonates are monophosphates (nucleotide analogs) requiring only two additional phosphates. Potency of the NAs in cell culture assays is partially influenced by the efficiency of the phosphorylation step. For example, entecavir is very efficiently converted to the triphosphate active substrate, a factor thought to be important in defining its greater potency in cell culture assays compared with the other NAs.

The resultant triphosphate active substrates act as competitive inhibitors of the viral DNA polymerase and reverse transcriptase by substituting for the native host nucleotides. Nucleos(t)ide analogs respective affinity to the "Palm" subdomain of the viral reverse transcriptase, the active site of nucleotide incorporation, also determines their potency, as determined by enzymic assays. Since they lack a 3'-hydroxyl group, incorporation of the NA into the elongating proviral DNA leads to chain termination. Though entecavir does have a 3'-hydroxyl moiety on its cyclopentyl group, it nevertheless halts elongation after a few nucleotide additions, hence still serving as a de facto chain terminator. While all the above-mentioned NAs obstruct the reverse transcription of pregenomic mRNA to the negative viral DNA strand as well as the next step of positive strand synthesis, entecavir also impedes the initial step of base priming by the polymerase. Though NAs slow or halt viral replication, they do not eradicate infected cells that already have proviral DNA integrated into their genome or prevent infection of susceptible cells by existing virus. Therefore, notwithstanding the rare event of a hepatitis B surface antigen (sAg) seroconversion by the host, they do not lead to a cure and have modest effects on HBsAg and eAg expression.

Nucleos(t)ide analogs discussed here have a very low affinity for human DNA polymerases including DNA polymerase-α and -β and mitochondrial DNA polymerase γ. Some NAs used in combination HIV therapy have a greater affinity to human mitochondrial DNA polymerase-γ and can lead to serious adverse events including lactic acidosis, pancytopenia, myopathy, peripheral neuropathy and pancreatitis. These side-effects are rarely seen with the NAs used to treat HBV infection as these agents have very low affinity for the human DNA polymerases and these effects are less common when used as monotherapy. An increased incidence of these complications has been shown to occur in HIV positive patients on antiretroviral therapy receiving ribavirin and interferon for HCV infection. A few cases of entecavir associated lactic acidosis have also been reported in patients with advanced liver disease.

Since NAs interfere with DNA replication there has been some concern that they may have an oncogenic effect. Entecavir has been associated with an increased risk of lung tumors in mice at doses 3–5 times greater than those use in humans. However this effect appears to be species specific. Doses 30–40 times the human equivalent have been shown to cause lung, brain and liver tumors in mice and rats.

Drug resistance

Mutations in the viral genome altering the nucleotide binding site on the reverse transcriptase confer drug resistance. The M204V substitution on the YMDD loop of the "palm" subdomain leads to lamivudine resistance by hampering this loop's anchoring of the triphosphate of the nucleotide and changing the pocket shape of the nucleotide binding site causing steric hindrance. This mutation is often accompanied by a compensatory adaptive mutation, L180M, restoring some viral replication fitness. It has full cross-resistance to the other structurally similar L-nucleoside analogs such as telbivudine and emtricitabine.

The M204V + L180M substitutions lead to partial cross-resistance with the structurally different entecavir. An additional substitution at T184, S202, or M250 that further restricts the active site pocket, is needed for full entecavir resistance. Hence complete entecavir resistance requires multiple viral mutations, explaining in part, why entecavir has such a high barrier to resistance. The A181V and N236T substitutions that lead to adefovir and tenofovir resistance alter how nucleotides fit into the active site pocket more indirectly by disrupting secondary stabilizing interactions.

Pharmacology

The NAs ease of use is attributable to some of their favorable pharmacological properties including generally high oral bioavailability, efficient cellular passive and active transport, longer cellular half-life of the active substrates, absence of cytochrome P450 metabolism, and renal excretion of unaltered drug (Table 10.2). The L-nucleosides and cyclopentane rings have high oral bioavailability, characteristically over 80%. The greater polarity of the nucleotide analogs due to their acyclic phosphonate group leads to poor oral bioavailability. This is circumvented by the development of diester prodrugs. Upon absorption, adefovir dipivoxil and tenofovir disoproxil are readily hydrolyzed by plasma and intestinal epithelium esterases to the active drug. In the case of adefovir, the liberation of the pivalic group contributes to the toxicity profile at higher doses.

The NAs generally have a volume of distribution equal to or exceeding total body water. They are scantly protein bound. Due to the efficient renal excretion of the parent drug, the plasma half-lives of the NAs discussed here are short, with the notable exception of entecavir. However, the intracellular phosphorylated active drug species have a longer half-life and consequently allow for once daily dosing.

The NAs do not undergo catabolism but are largely excreted unchanged by the kidney. As a result they are associated with only few drug–drug interactions. Furthermore, NAs should be dose adjusted in renal but not liver failure. Renal excretion occurs through both glomerular filtration and tubular excretion. The acyclic phosphonates (adefovir and tenofovir) undergo efficient transport at the renal proximal tubules by organic anion transporter (hOAT) and their accumulation there explains the associated renal toxicity. In addition, there may be competition for excretion with other drug substrates of hOAT, such as some protease inhibitors, resulting in drug–drug interaction.

Table 10.2 Pharmacokinetic properties of NAs

Drug	Telbivudine	Lamivudine	Adefovir	Tenofovir	Entecavir	Ribavirin
Bioavailability	Unknown	82–87%	59%	25% (40% with food)	100%	64%
Effect of food on bioavailability	None	None	None	Increased (take with meal)	Decreased (take fasting)	Increased (take with meal)
Volume of distribution	Extensive	0.9–1.7 L/kg	0.4 L/Kg	1.2–1.3L/kg	Extensive (>TBW)[†]	10 L/kg
Protein binding	3%	<36%	<4%	<7%	13%	None
Plasma $t_{1/2}$ (cellular $t_{1/2}$) in hours	40–49	3–7 (12–18)	5–7.5 (16–18)	14–17 (>49)	128–149	200–300
Elimination	Renal excretion	Renal excretion	Renal excretion	Renal excretion	Renal excretion	Hepatic metabolism + renal excretion

[†]TBW=total body water.

Clinical effectiveness

Management decisions in chronic hepatitis B are complex given that current treatments do not eradicate the infection. Treatment, once begun, is largely indefinite and carries the goals of preventing progression to cirrhosis and liver failure as well as lowering the incidence of hepatocellular cancer. Initiation of treatment must be weighed against the risk of adverse events, cost, risk of viral resistance and compliance with long term treatment. Elevation in alanine aminotransferase (ALT), viral load and evidence of progressive liver disease are the best prognosticators and are the key factor used in the current guidelines for treatment. Age, presence of cirrhosis, family history of hepatocellular carcinoma (HCC), comorbid disease, as well as family planning (*future pregnancy*) must also be weighed in the decision to commence treatment as well as affecting the choice of agent. Likelihood of response to treatment, which both viral load and ALT may predict, is also considered. A comprehensive review of chronic hepatitis B management is beyond the scope of this chapter. A brief summary of our approach, based on current guidelines is summarized in Figure 10.1. Treatment is also indicated in patients with HBV

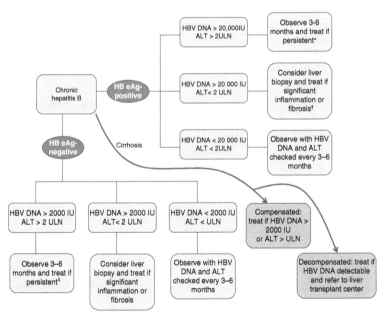

*Oral Antiviral (NAs) up to 6 month after seroconversion and no less than 1 year total or in select patients may consider PegINF-α for 48 weeks.
†May consider obtaining liver biopsy to guide treatment, especially if age>40, ALT > ULN, or family history HCC.
‡End point not defined.

Figure 10.1 Chronic hepatitis B treatment algorithm. IU, international units; ULN, upper limit of normal.

markers post liver transplantation, in selected patients with severe acute hepatitis B infection, and for the prevention of HBV reactivation with immunosuppressive chemotherapy (e.g., rituximab). Treatment should also be considered in the last trimester of pregnancy for prevention of vertical transmission.

Based on their clinical efficacy and high barrier to resistance entecavir and tenofovir are the NAs of first choice once a decision to treat is made. The choice as to which of these drugs should be used is based on the risk of drug toxicities in an individual patient as well as prior NA exposure/resistance. The initial goals of therapy are to achieve complete viral suppression, undetectable HBV DNA levels with normalization of liver blood tests. Viral suppression is associated with improved clinical outcomes, including a reduced risk of hepatocellular carcinoma and in some patients regression of liver fibrosis, even resolution of cirrhosis has been described. End-points for treatment are more difficult. The ultimate end-point is HBsAg seroconversion, but this is achieved in only a tiny proportion of patients even with long-term treatment. In HBeAg positive patients, HBeAg seroconversion is often used as the end-point but treatment should be continued for 6–12 months after seroconversion to reduce the risk of viral relapse, and long-term monitoring is required. In HBeAg negative patients there is no clear end-point and therapy should probably be continued indefinitely. Measurement of HBsAg levels is currently being evaluated as a means to identify patients in whom treatment can be stopped. These markers of therapy outcomes including biochemical (ALT) normalization, virologic suppression (nondetectable viral DNA), eAg seroconversion, sAg loss along with the rate of viral resistance are outlined in Table 10.3A and 10.3B for the respective NAs.

The major concern with long-term antiviral therapy is the development of viral breakthrough and viral resistance. Complete viral suppression and good long-term compliance minimizes the risk of resistance. Once viral resistance occurs salvage therapy should be implemented. Addition, rather than substitution, is preferred. When resistance to a nucleoside analog such as lamivudine occurs, addition of a nucleotide analog such as tenofovir is indicated, and vice versa. The development of viral resistance or sudden discontinuation of treatment can lead to life-threatening flares of hepatitis B. Close monitoring for viral resistance or viral flares after stopping treatment is therefore recommended.

Pregnancy

Possible teratogenicity of NAs should be discussed with women of child bearing age prior to initiation of treatment for CHB. Women who are planning on starting a family and who have mild liver disease may choose to postpone treatment. Women already on CHB treatment who become pregnant may elect to switch NA to tenofovir or lamivudine, which have known better safety profiles in this setting. Antiviral treatment for prophylaxis of perinatal transmission should be considered in women with CHB who reach the third trimester with a high viral load, greater than 2×10^7 International Units (or in women with previous child with HBsAg positivity, greater than 2×10^6 International Units).

HIV
Patients with HIV/HBV co-infection are at risk for an accelerated course of liver disease including increased incidence of HCC and progression to cirrhosis. Use of agent(s) with dual activity such as tenofovir plus emtricitabine as part of a full HIV antiretroviral therapy is advised.

Patients receiving immunosuppressive therapy
HBsAg positive patients who are expected to receive immunosuppressive therapy of a finite duration should receive prophylactic antiviral therapy. Choice of agent and duration is dependent on baseline HBV DNA level and anticipated duration of immunosuppressive treatment.

Nucleoside analogs

The pharmacology, clinical efficacy, side-effect and resistance profiles of each of the NA are summarized in Tables 10.2, 10.3 and 10.4.

Lamivudine
Lamivudine, an enantiomer of 2, 3 thiacytidine, is a nucleoside analog with activity against both HIV and HBV polymerases. High rates of resistance with long-term use, and the fact that resistance to lamivudine induces complete or partial resistance to other nucleoside analogs has limited its use, and as a result lamivudine is no longer considered a first-line agent for the treatment of chronic hepatitis B. However, its excellent safety profile, as well as long-term experience means that it may still have a role in specific situations, such as prevention of vertical transmission, prevention of HBV reactivation and occasionally in acute hepatitis B. Lamivudine resistant mutants may be treated with nucleotide analogs or high-dose entecavir. Viral mutations associated with lamivudine resistance occur in the YMDD motif and include M204V/I + L180M. These mutations are associated with resistance to other L-nucleoside analogs as well as relative resistance to entecavir. The L-nucleoside analogs can also select for the A181T/V mutation which also confers resistance to the nucleotide analogs (adefovir and tenofovir) hence giving rise to a multi-resistant virus.

Table 10.3A NAs' clinical effectiveness for eAg-positive CHB

Treatment response at 48-52 weeks	Lamivudine	Telbivudine	Entecavir	Adefovir	Tenofovir
Undetectable HBV DNA at 48–52 weeks %	36–44	60	67	13–21	76
HBeAg SC % [+]	16–21	22	21	12–18	21
HBsAg loss %	<1	<1	2	0	3
Genotypic resistance %	27	4.4	0	0	0
Response to extended treatment	At 2 years 39% undetectable DNA; at 3 years 47% eAg SC at 5 years 65% resistance.	At 4 years 79% undetectable DNA; at 4 years 42% eAg SC at 2 years 21% resistance.	At 5 years 94% undetectable DNA, 41% eAg SC, 1.2% resistance.	At 5 years 39% undetectable DNA, 48% eAg SC, and 42% resistance.	At 5 years 65% undetectable DNA; at 4 years 31% eAg SC at 5 years no resistance.

[+]SC = seroconversion.

Source: Scaglione SJ, Lok ASF (2012). Reproduced with permission of Elsevier.

Table 10.3B NAs' clinical effectiveness for eAg-negative CHB

Treatment Response at 48–52 weeks	Lamivudine	Telbivudine	Entecavir	Adefovir	Tenofovir
Undetectable HBV DNA at 48–52 weeks %	60–73	88	90	51	93
HBsAg loss %	<1	<1	<1	0	0
Genotypic resistance %	23	2.7	0.2	0	0
Response to extended treatment	At 4 years 6% undetectable DNA; at 5 years 70–80% resistance.	At 4 years 84% undetectable DNA; at 2 years 8.6% resistance.	Not available	At 5 years 67% undetectable DNA and 29% resistance.	At 5 years 83% undetectable DNA and no resistance.

Source: Scaglione SJ, Lok ASF (2012). Reproduced with permission of Elsevier.

Table 10.4 NAs' side effect profile and parameters to monitor

Drug	Side effects	Monitor: For all chronic hepatitis B NA treatment follow HBV DNA, LFTs* every 3–6 months and at longer intervals eAg and sAg
Lamivudine	Gastrointestinal symptoms (abdominal pain, diarrhea, nausea, vomiting), headaches, myalgia, stomatitis, pancreatitis, lactic acidosis, rash	BMP and CBC every 3–6 months, FBG every 6 months, FLP annually, UA annually
Telbivudine	Gastrointestinal symptoms (abdominal pain, diarrhea, nausea, vomiting), headache, myopathy, peripheral neuropathy, lactic acidosis	BMP and CBC every 3–6 months, creatine kinase, UA annually
Adefovir	Nephrotoxicity, lactic acidosis, osteopenia, headache, gastrointestinal (abdominal pain, diarrhea), hematuria	Bone Marrow Density with DEXA BMP† and CBC every 3–6 months, FBG every 6 months, FLP annually; UA annually Serum phosphorus in patients with or at risk for renal impairment
Tenofovir	Fanconi syndrome, nephrotoxicity, rash, osteopenia, gastrointestinal (abdominal pain, diarrhea)	Bone marrow density with DEXA BMP† and CBC every 3–6 months, FBG every 6 months, FLP annually; UA annually Serum phosphorus in patients with or at risk for renal impairment
Entecavir	Gastrointestinal (abdominal pain, diarrhea, nausea), headache, lactic acidosis, hematuria	BMP and CBC every 3–6 months
Ribavirin	Anemia, leukopenia, thrombocytopenia, nausea, abdominal pain, anorexia, rash, alopecia, pruritus, insomnia, dyspnea, cough	During hepatitis C therapy follow viral RNA levels at intervals per guidelines and hepatic function. CBC and BMP at week 2 and 4 of therapy and at least every 4 weeks thereafter. TSH at initiation of therapy and week 12 Pregnancy test monthly in women of childbearing age

*BMP, basic metabolic panel; CBC, complete blood count; FBG, fasting blood glucose; FLP, fasting lipid profile; LFT, liver function tests; UA, urinalysis.
†In patients with renal impairment consider shorter intervals for UA (6 months) and BMP (3 months).

Telbivudine

Telbivudine is a synthetic thymidine analog with activity against HBV DNA polymerase. Lamivudine resistance (M204V/I + L180M) confers a marked reduction in susceptibility to telbivudine and modest reduction in sensitivity to telbivudine has been seen in association with adefovir resistant (A181V, A181S and A181T) mutants. Telbivudine retains activity against the isolated lamivudine M204V mutant as well as the adefovir N236T mutant. Resistance to telbivudine occurs in up to 25% of patients after 2 years of therapy. For this reason, as well as the availability of better alternatives, telbivudine is not considered a first line agent for the treatment of chronic hepatitis B. Side effects include: myopathy, increase in creatine kinase levels, nausea, and diarrhea.

Emtricitabine

Structurally similar to lamivudine, emtricitabine is potent against both HBV and HIV but likewise suffers from high rate of HBV resistance. It is available as Truvada, a combination pill with the nucleotide analog, Tenofovir. Truvada may provide a convenient option for HIV/HBV coinfected patients or those with lamivudine resistant HBV.

Entecavir

Entecavir is a guanosine analog with specific activity against HBV DNA polymerase. Entecavir is well absorbed from the GI tract, but absorption is reduced by administration with food, so it is recommended that the drug be taken on an empty stomach. Entecavir is a highly potent inhibitor of HBV DNA polymerase, but lamivudine resistant mutants are associated with an 8-30 fold reduction in entecavir susceptibility. Full entecavir resistance requires multiple mutations. In addition to the lamivudine resistance mutations M204V and L180M, a mutation of at least one of the following positions I169T, T184G, S202I or M250V is required for entecavir resistance. Higher doses of entecavir are recommended in patients with lamivudine resistant strains of HBV. Entecavir when administered to patients with HIV coinfection has been shown to select for HIV mutants and to cause partial suppression of HIV RNA levels. For this reason, entecavir should not be administered to HIV positive patients who are not on antiretroviral therapy. Entecavir is generally well tolerated with a few patients reporting headache, fatigue, nausea and abdominal pain. Due to its high potency and high threshold for genotypic resistance, entecavir is a first line therapy. A few cases of lactic acidosis have been reported in patients with advanced liver disease.

Nucleotide analogs

Adefovir

Adefovir Dipivoxil is a diester prodrug of adefovir, an adenosine nucleotide analog. The diester prodrug is required to enhance absorption. It is rapidly hydrolyzed in the blood and intestine to adefovir. Adefovir causes dose dependent tubular dysfunction that can result in a Fanconi like syndrome with increases in creatinine, proteinuria, hypophosphatemia and glycosuria. However these side-effects are unusual at the low doses (10 mg daily) used in HBV infection. Resistance to adefovir does occur with long-term use but most adefovir resistant strains retain sensitivity to nucleoside analogs. Most lamivudine resistant strains are sensitive to adefovir. The adefovir resistant mutations, N236T and A181T/V are associated with intermediate resistance to tenofovir. Furthermore as mentioned above the A181T/V mutation confers partial or complete resistance to the L-nucleoside analogs. The lower rates of resistance and increased clinical efficacy of tenofovir has meant that this drug has largely supplanted adefovir as a first line agent.

Tenofovir

Tenofovir is an adenosine nucleotide analog, akin to Adefovir, with low cross resistance to lamivudine resistant HBV. Tenofovir is presented as the disoproxil prodrug to facilitate absorption which can be further enhanced by being taken with a high fat meal, though this is not generally recommended. Tenofovir is generally well tolerated with few side-effects the most common being diarrhea, abdominal pain, nausea, headache and generalized weakness. A few cases of Fanconi-like syndrome have been reported and as a result this agent should be used with caution in patients with renal impairment. Routine monitoring should include measurement of serum creatinine and phosphate levels as well as urinalysis. Tenofovir has also been associated with decreased bone mineral density, an issue primarily reported in patients with HIV infection receiving multiple agents. However, monitoring of bone density and treatment with vitamin D and calcium should be considered in susceptible individuals. Tenofovir's higher potency and very high threshold for genotypic resistance have placed it as a first-line agent and it has largely superseded adefovir for the treatment of hepatitis B. Adefovir resistant mutants retain some, though often reduced, sensitivity to tenofovir.

Ribavirin

A nucleoside analog of guanosine, ribavirin is unique in its activity against a wide range of DNA and RNA viruses. It has taken a prominent role in chronic hepatitis C (CHC) treatment in combination with interferon and protease inhibitors, where it has led to overall sustain virologic response of nearly 70%. It has also been approved in aerosolized form for the treatment of RSV bronchiolitis and pneumonia. Additionally, it has been used in the treatment of a variety of hemorrhagic fevers, including most notably Lassa fever.

This wide range of viral activity is likely explained by the multi-faceted mechanism of action of ribavirin which is incompletely understood. The following three mechanisms contributed to its antiviral activity. First, it alters intracellular guanosine triphosphate pools by inhibiting cellular inosine monophosphate dehydrogenase. Second, it may interfere with 5′ capping of viral mRNA disrupting translation. Lastly, as other NAs, it inhibits viral polymerases. During hepatitis C therapy, it has been suggested that ribavirin mainly acts as a viral mutagen leading to error catastrophe during viral replication. In addition, ribavirin enhances the expression of INF-stimulated response genes hence synergizing Peg-INF treatment.

Ribavirin's pharmacokinetic properties, listed in Table 10.2, are notable for its good oral bioavailability, large volume of distribution, and long plasma half-life. Unlike the above-mentioned NAs, ribavirin undergoes significant hepatic metabolism, encompassing deribosylation and hydrolysis. Renal excretion still plays a key role in clearance.

The principle adverse event associated with ribavirin administration is anemia, driven by both hemolysis as well as bone marrow suppression. Caution should be exercised in the patient at a baseline risk for anemia, such as those with hemoglobinopathies, or patients with underlying medical conditions in which anemia may lead to complications, such as cardiovascular disease. It should be emphasized that ribavirin is pregnancy category X due to its teratogenic and embryotoxic properties and is contraindicated in both pregnant women and their male partners. A washout period of 6 months is required after chronic treatment before conception.

Summary

- Nucleos(t)ide analogs serve as potent oral antivirals by competitively inhibiting viral DNA polymerase as well as leading to chain termination.
- The NAs generally have high oral bioavailability and a longer intracellular half-life allowing daily dosing.
- The NAs low affinity for human nuclear or mitochondrial DNA polymerase explains why mitochondria toxicity, such as lactic acidosis, rarely occurs and tumorgenicity is not observed.

- Nucleos(t)ide analogs primarily undergo renal excretion unchanged. The absence of other catabolism explains the low rate of drug–drug interactions. Renal toxicity, however, is seen in some.
- The NAs are highly potent against chronic hepatitis B, but development of drug resistance may hamper long-term use. The low rate of drug resistance observed with entecavir and tenofovir has advanced them as first-line agents.
- The nucleoside analogs, including lamivudine and entecavir, have low cross-resistance activity with the nucleotide analogs, adefovir and tenofovir. A nucleotide analog can be added when resistance to a nucleoside analog occurs during treatment, and vice versa.
- As NAs do not eradicate the hepatitis B infection, they generally obligate lifelong treatment. Treatment is aimed at reducing the progression to cirrhosis and incidence of hepatocellular cancer.
- Nucleos(t)ide analogs are very well tolerated and have a minimal side effect profile.
- Ribavirin, a nucleoside analog, has a more complex mechanism which is not well understood but which leads to a wider range of antiviral activity. Its primary use is in combination with interferon for treatment of chronic hepatitis C.

Recommended reading

Acosta EP, Flexner C (2011) Antiviral agents (nonretroviral). In: LL Brunton, BA Chabner, BC Knollmann (eds.), *Goodman & Gilman's The Pharmacological Basis of Therapeutics*. 12th edn. New York: McGraw-Hill, Chapter 58.
  This chapter from a pharmacology text provides an excellent starting point in understanding the mechanism and pharmacology of the nucleos(t)ides.
Brillanti S, Mazzella G, Roda E. (2011) Ribavirin for chronic hepatitis C: And the mystery goes on. *Digestive and Liver Disease* **43**(6): 425–30.
Chang T, Gish RG, de Man R, *et al.* (2006) A comparison of entecavir and lamivudine for HBeAg-positive chronic hepatitis B. *N Engl J Med* **354**(10): 1001–10.
Dienstag JL, Schiff ER, Wright TL, *et al.* (1999) Lamivudine as initial treatment for chronic hepatitis B in the united states. *N Engl J Med.* **341**(17): 1256–63.
Flexner C (2011) Antiretroviral agents and treatment of HIV Infection In: LL Brunton, BA Chabner, BC Knollmann (eds.), *Goodman & Gilman's The Pharmacological Basis of Therapeutics*. 12th edn. New York: McGraw-Hill, Chapter 59.
Gallant JE, Moore RD (2009) Renal function with use of a tenofovir-containing initial antiretroviral regimen. *AIDS*, **23**: 1971–5.
Ghany MG, Nelson DR, Strader DB, Thomas DL, Seeff LB (2011) An update on treatment of genotype 1 chronic hepatitis C virus infection: 2011 practice guideline by the american association for the study of liver diseases. *Hepatology.* **54**(4): 1433–44.
Gish RG, Lok AS, Chang T, *et al.* (2007) Entecavir therapy for up to 96 weeks in patients with HBeAg-positive chronic hepatitis B. *Gastroenterology.* **133**(5): 1437–44.

Hynicka LM, Yunker N, Patel PH (2010) A review of oral antiretroviral therapy for the treatment of chronic hepatitis B. *The Annals of Pharmacotherapy.* **44**(7): 1271–86.
An excellent review article of nucleos(t)ides with tables summarizing the important trials.
Lange CM, Bojunga J, Hofmann WP, *et al.* (2009) Severe lactic acidosis during treatment of chronic hepatitis B with entecavir in patients with impaired liver function. *Hepatology* **50**(6): 2001–6.
Langley DR, Walsh AW, Baldick CJ, *et al.* (2007) Inhibition of hepatitis B virus polymerase by entecavir. *Journal of Virology* Apr.; **81**(8): 3992–4001.
A good review of the molecular mechanism of nucleoside analog inhibition of DNA polymerase.
Lok AS, Trinh H, Carosi G, *et al.* (2012) Efficacy of entecavir with or without tenofovir disoproxil fumarate for nucleos(t)ide-naïve patients with chronic hepatitis B. *Gastroenterology* **143**(3): 619–28.
Lok ASF, McMahon BJ (2009) Chronic hepatitis B: Update 2009. *Hepatology* **50**(3): 661–2.
AASLD comprehensive guidelines for treatment of Hepatitis B.
Petersen J, Ratziu V, Buti M, *et al.* (2012) Entecavir plus tenofovir combination as rescue therapy in pre-treated chronic hepatitis B patients: An international multicenter cohort study. *J Hepatol* **56**(3): 520–6.
Ray SA, Hitchcock MJM (2009) Metabolism of antiviral nucleosides and nucleotides. In: RL LaFemina (ed.), *Antiviral Research: Strategies in Antiviral Drug Discovery.* Washington, DC, USA: ASM Press, Chapter 17.
Scaglione SJ, Lok ASF (2012) Effectiveness of hepatitis B treatment in clinical practice. *Gastroenterology.* **142**(6): 1360–8.
A recent review giving an updated perspective on hepatitis B treatment.
Severini A, Liu XY, Wilson JS, Tyrrell D (1995) Mechanism of inhibition of duck hepatitis B virus polymerase by (-)-beta-L-2′, 3′-dideoxy-3′-thiacytidine. *Antimicrob Agents Chemother* **39**(7): 1430–5.
Suh DJ, Um SH, Herrmann E, *et al.* (2010) Early viral kinetics of telbivudine and entecavir: Results of a 12-week randomized exploratory study with patients with HBeAg-positive chronic hepatitis B. *Antimicrobial Agents and Chemotherapy* Mar.; **54**(3): 1242–7.
Describes the short-term virological kinetics of entecavir vs telbivudine with good references to similar questions regarding other nucleos(t)ides.
Wilber R, Kreter B, Bifano M, Danetz S, Lehman-McKeeman L, Tenney DJ, Meanwell N, Zahler R, Brett-Smith H (2011) Discovery and development of entecavir. In: WM Kazmierski (ed.), *Antiviral Drugs: From Basic Discovery through Clinical Trials.* Hoboken, NJ, USA: John Wiley ^& Sons, Inc, Chapter 28.
A thoughtful narrative of the development of a nucleoside antiviral agents that provides insight on the discovery and pharmacology of these agents.

CHAPTER 11
Ursodeoxycholic acid, chelating agents, and zinc in the treatment of metabolic liver diseases

Andrew K. Burroughs and James S. Dooley
University College London, London, UK

Ursodeoxycholic acid

Introduction

Ursodeoxycholic acid (UDCA), also known as ursodiol, is a secondary bile acid, which is physiologically the by-product of intestinal bacteria acting on primary bile acids secreted by the liver into the biliary system and the gut.

Pharmacologically, UDCA is chemically synthesized and is licensed in the treatment of cholesterol-rich gallstones, primary biliary cirrhosis, and the prophylaxis of gallstone formation in patients undergoing rapid weight loss.

UDCA is also used to treat cholestasis of pregnancy, primary sclerosing cholangitis and other cholestatic diseases, such as the liver disease of cystic fibrosis and progressive familial intrahepatic cholestasis. It is also used as a general " hepatoprotective," as it can improve abnormal liver function tests nonspecifically, as in chronic hepatitis C.

Commercial preparations of UDCA are shown in Table 11.1.

Pharmacology

UCDA suppresses hepatic synthesis and secretion of cholesterol and inhibits intestinal absorption of cholesterol. It is rapidly absorbed from the GI tract and is 90% bioavailable. It is 96–98% protein-bound in plasma, and undergoes entero-hepatic recycling. In the liver, it is partly conjugated before excretion into the bile. In the gut, a small amount of both free and conjugated UDCA is metabolized by bacteria (7α dehydroxylation) to lithocholic acid. The latter is mainly excreted in feces but

Pocket Guide to Gastrointestinal Drugs, Edited by M. Michael Wolfe and Robert C. Lowe. © 2014 John Wiley & Sons, Ltd. Published 2014 by John Wiley & Sons, Ltd.

Table 11.1 Commercial names for UCDA

Trade name	Manufacturer
Actibile	Albert David
Actigall	Axcan/Watson Pharmaceuticals
Analiv	Systopic Labs.(P)
BILIVER	Sedico
Deursil	Torrinomedica
Dulic	Edura Pharmaceuticals
Egyurso	Egyphar
Golbi	Arron (Intas Pharm.)
Intraliv	Intra Labs India
Livokind	Mankind Pharm.
Udcoliv	Marc Laboratories
Udebile	Life Medicare
Udihep (Forte)	Win Medicare
Udilite	Aqcor Drug
Udiliv	Solvay Pharma India
Udkare	Nitro Cardineur
Udoxyl	Ind Swift
Udxic	Zee Laboratories
Urchil (Forte)	Sioux Laboratories
Urdiogem	Alembic Chemical Works
URS	Synokem Pharmaceuticals
Urso	Curewell Drugs & Pharm.
Urso Forte	Aptalis
Ursocol (SR)	Sun Pharm. Industries
Ursodil	German Remedies
Ursodox (SR)	Signova Pharma
Ursofalk	Falk Pharmaceuticals
Ursohep	Adroit Lifescience
Ursol	Corona Remedies
Ursolic	Stadmed
Ursoliv	Durga Pharma
Ursoriv	East Africa
Ursosan	Pro Medics

20% is absorbed and sulphated by the liver. Excretion of UDCA conjugates is almost 100% fecal.

With continued administration, UDCA concentrations in bile reach a steady state in approximately 3 weeks. UDCA solubilizes the normally insoluble cholesterol in normal bile, and also leads to dispersion of cholesterol as liquid crystals. Thus, even though administration of high doses (e.g., 15–18 mg/kg/day) does not result in concentrating UDCA to more than 60% of the total bile acid pool, UDCA-rich bile effectively solubilizes cholesterol and increases the concentration level at which saturation of cholesterol occurs.

Thus, the bile of patients with gallstones treated with UCDA changes from cholesterol-precipitating to cholesterol-solubilizing, which facilitates cholesterol stone dissolution. UDCA competes with endogenous bile acids for absorption in the terminal ileum, interrupting their enterohepatic circulation and thereby increasing their elimination in feces.

When UDCA is discontinued, its concentration in bile falls rapidly to about 5–10% of its steady-state level after about 1 week.

In cholestatic liver disease or injury, the therapeutic action of UDCA is based on experimental evidence. There are 3 major mechanisms of action: (1) protection against the cytotoxicity of hydrophobic bile acids by changing the composition of mixed phospholipid-rich micelles in bile, thus reducing bile acid cytotoxic effects on the cholangiocytes; (2) stimulation of hepatobiliary secretion by activating and/or inserting transporter molecules (such as MRP2) into the canalicular membrane of the hepatocyte; and (3) protection of hepatocytes against bile acid-induced apoptosis.

Drug interactions
The effectiveness of UDCA is reduced with co-administration of cholestyramine, charcoal and aluminium-based antacids. Oestrogens and clofibrate increase cholesterol elimination in bile and may also decrease the effectiveness of UCDA. Administration of UCDA reduces the effectiveness of dapsone and may increase concentrations in blood of cyclosporine, and nitrendipine.

Licensed therapeutic indications
Gallstone dissolution
This indication is for cholesterol-rich gallstones (ie radiolucent stones without calcium deposits), in patients with a functioning gall bladder. UCDA is given as 6–12 mg/Kg/day orally as a single dose or 2–3 divided doses. It is continued for 3–4 months after ultrasound evidence of dissolution of stones. With 10 mg/kg/day dosing, complete stone dissolution occurs in about 30% of patients with uncalcified gallstones less

than 20 mm in maximal diameter, treated for up to 2 years. Larger diameter stones are unlikely to dissolve while smaller stones have increased chances of dissolution. If there are floating or floatable stones (indicating a high cholesterol content), gallstone dissolution is increased up to 50%.

However, stone recurrence after dissolution occurs in 30–50% within 5 years of stopping UDCA, and continued ultrasound monitoring is necessary after therapy.

Gallstone prevention
Prophylaxis of gallstone formation is indicated in obese patients undergoing rapid weight loss. The dose of UDCA for this indication is 300mg twice a day, as larger doses do not have a greater preventative effect. Studies demonstrate that between 6% and 9% of UDCA-treated patients developed gall stones compared to 23% in placebo groups despite similar loss in weight in both groups.

Primary biliary cirrhosis (PBC)
In 2 meta-analyses, which included a wide spectrum of severity of PBC from mild to moderate/severe, the use of UDCA (13–15 mg/Kg/day) did not decrease mortality, or the rate of liver transplantation. However, in early PBC there is nonrandomized evidence that sustained biochemical amelioration of abnormal liver function tests after one year of UDCA (13–15 mg/kg) administration (i.e., a reduction of alkaline phosphatase <3x the upper limit of the normal range, with a total serum bilirubin of 1 mg/dl or less, together with a serum aspartate transaminase 2 times the upper limit of normal) significantly improved 10-year transplantation free survival.This evidence is the basis for the licence in PBC. If the biochemical parameters do not reach the "response" criteria thresholds it is likely that further UDCA may not be effective, but stopping rules have not been formally evaluated for biochemical nonresponders.

Special circumstances
Pregnancy
UCDA has a category B rating from the US FDA. However, UDCA is used to treat cholestasis of pregnancy, which develops in the late 2nd and 3rd trimesters, avoiding the potentially higher-risk period for teratogenicity. There are no attributable reports of teratogenicity with UDCA.

A meta analysis of 9 randomized studies showed that UCDA (dose range from 600 mg to 1000 mg/day) was significantly associated with total resolution of pruritus, normalization of alanine aminotransferase levels, fewer premature births, and a decreased need for neonatal intensive care. The authors recommended UDCA as first-line therapy for cholestasis of pregnancy up to the time of delivery. A recent randomized study confirmed a reduction in pruritus but less than that perceived a priori to be clinically important by both patients and clinicians; planned early delivery did not increase Caesarean section rates.The safety of UDCA during lactation has not been established, so UDCA should be discontinued after delivery.

Primary sclerosing cholangitis (PSC)
As UDCA ameliorates abnormalities of liver function tests, it is used to treat PSC, but there has been no evidence of clinical effectiveness with standard dosing as for PBC. Its therapeutic effectiveness has been further debated since a randomized trial of higher dose (28–30 mg/Kg/day) in PSC demonstrated, despite significant improvement of liver function tests as in PBC, an adjusted increased risk (hazard ratio 2.1) of death, liver transplantation, and worsening MELD score There were also more adverse events in UCDA-treated patients. This trial has changed the perception of clinicians that UCDA is completely safe in patients with chronic liver disease. Thus, patients with PSC should not be given more than 15 mg/Kg/day of UDCA outside of clinical trials.

Use in children
The safety and effectiveness of UCDA in children has not been established; the recommended dose is 10–15 mg/Kg/day in 2–3 divided doses.

Adverse reactions
UDCA can cause diarrhea, pruritus, nausea, vomiting, and gallstone calcification. In randomized trials for treatment or prevention of gallstones there were no significant differences in side effects compared to placebo, whereas in treatment of cholestatic liver diseases, UDCA resulted in more side effects than placebo or no treatment. There have been no reported fatalities attributable to use of UCDA. Neither accidental nor intentional overdosing with UCDA has been reported: doses in the range of 16–20 mg/kg/day have been tolerated for 6–37 months without symptoms in patients treated for gallstones.

Contraindications for the use of UDCA are shown in Table 11.2.

Table 11.2 Contraindications for use of UCDA

Calcified and pigment gall stones
Radio-opaque gall stones
Severe chronic liver disease
First trimester of pregnancy
High dose (28–30 mg/Kg/day) in primary sclerosing cholangitis

Treatment of copper overload

Introduction

Wilson's disease is an autosomal recessive condition in which mutations in the ATP7B gene lead to dysfunction of an intracellular copper transporter. This results in accumulation of copper in hepatocytes due to a failure of biliary excretion and subsequent hepatic damage leading to a range of liver presentations. Accumulation of copper in the brain, and particularly the basal ganglia, leads to neuropsychiatric disease. Other organs may also be affected, including the kidney. Guidelines for diagnosis and management have been published in the USA and Europe, and these and other reviews give comprehensive details regarding the management of this condition and the choice of medications to be used.

The features of Wilson's disease were first collated in Samuel Alexander Kinnier Wilson's seminal paper in 1912 (Wilson, 1912). The role of copper was appreciated in the 1940s and the first treatment used to remove copper was dimercaprol (British anti-Lewisite), which had to be administered by intramuscular injection.

The oral copper chelators, penicillamine and trientine, were developed by Dr John Walshe, who published on the chelating effect of penicillamine in 1956; this agent has been the mainstay of treatment for over 50 years. Dr Walshe later introduced trientine hydrochloride,which initially was used as an alternative when penicillamine could not be used, but more recently has become, for some, an acceptable primary therapy.

Oral copper chelators exert their effect by promoting the urinary excretion of copper. Zinc compounds, when given orally, induce intestinal metalloproteins that reduce copper absorption from the gut. Such treatment was described by Schouwink in the early 1960s, and extended subsequently by Hoogenraad and, in a series of publications, Brewer. Negative copper balance takes longer to achieve with zinc than with chelators and guidelines recommend that initial treatment of patients presenting with symptomatic disease should include a chelating agent. Once clinical improvement has occurred and copper status optimized, a maintenance phase is entered. Some specialists will then reduce the dose of chelator, while others will use zinc therapy to control copper balance.

Wilson's disease is rare and therefore in order to optimize management, manage the side effects of medication, best monitor copper parameters, and give appropriate advice to patients and families, it is best to seek advice from a centre with experience in treating this disorder. Patient-led associations also provide a valuable resource of information and contact for patients. Treatment for Wilson's Disease is lifelong, unless liver transplantation is performed, which corrects the metabolic abnormality and "cures" the disease.

The trade names of some of the currently available medications are shown in Table 11.3.

Table 11.3 Generic and trade names of medications

Generic name	Trade name/other
Penicillamine	Cuprimine (ATON); Depen (MEDA)
Trientine	Trientine (UNIVAR); Syprine (ATON)
Zinc acetate	Wilzin (ORPHAN EUROPE); Galzin (TEVA)

Pharmacology

Penicillamine

Penicillamine is derived from the amino acid cysteine with the substitution of two methyl groups on the sulfhydryl-containing side chain; the free sulphydryl group acts as a copper chelator. Absorption from the gastrointestinal tract is rapid, but if taken with food, absorption is reduced by approximately 50%. Circulating penicillamine is predominantly bound to plasma proteins (80%). More than 80% of the penicillamine is excreted in the urine, with an excretion half life of 1.7–7 hrs. Thus, penicillamine chelates copper which is excreted with the drug in urine. In addition, penicillamine is an inducer of metallothionein, a protein rich in cysteine that is an endogenous chelator of metals.

Penicillamine should be taken on an empty stomach, one hour before (preferable) or two hours after eating, since food significantly reduces the amount of drug absorbed. The maximum dose is 1000–1500 mg/day in two to four divided doses. To reduce the risk of adverse effects (see below) penicillamine should be introduced gradually; for example, begin with 250–500 mg/day (125–250 mg/day if neurological disease), increasing by 250 mg/day every 4–7 days to reach the target dose over a few weeks.

Once clinical improvement has been achieved and copper studies are optimized, the dose of chelator is reduced to approximately 750–1000 mg/day.

Drug interactions. Antacids are stated to reduce absorption of penicillamine, as may oral iron salts. Zinc compounds should not be taken with penicillamine as each may attenuate the effect of the other agent. Penicillamine may decrease the plasma concentration of digoxin. The British National Formulary notes a possible increase in nephrotoxicity when penicillamine is given with NSAIDs, and stipulates avoidance of concomitant use of penicillamine and the antipsychotic clozapine because of the particular risk of agranulocytosis with this combination.

Penicillamine can affect pyridoxine metabolism and guidelines recommend that pyridoxine (vitamin B6) should be coadministered (25–50 mg/day). Deficiency in pyridoxine could particularly affect children, pregnant women, and those with malnutrition or an intercurrent illness.

Trientine hydrochloride

Trientine, a polyamine, chelates copper by forming stable complexes with the four nitrogens in a planar ring. It needs to be stored in the cold to prevent deterioration. There appears to be little information on the pharmacokinetics of trientine, but it is poorly absorbed, with approximately 1% of administered drug appearing in urine (8% of the metabolite acetyltrien). It is not clear whether it is a more or less potent chelator than penicillamine, and whether these two chelators remove copper from different pools.

As in the case of penicillamine, trientine should be taken on an empty stomach, one hour before or two hours after eating. The initial dose in guidelines is 750–1500 mg/day in two to three divided doses. Typical doses vary between publications, and the situation is complicated by different brands containing a different milligram content per individual preparation. A dose of 20 mg/kg/day has been suggested; one guideline refers to typical initial doses being between 900–2700 mg/day. Thus dosage will be determined by the weight of the patient and the clinical scenario, copper studies and the response to treatment.

As with penicillamine, once clinical improvement has been achieved and copper studies are optimized, the dose of trientine is reduced according to the clinical and metabolic status, with continued close monitoring.

Drug interactions. As with penicillamine, zinc should be administered well separated from trientine, since they reduce each others' action. Antacids may decrease the absorption of trientine, and trientine has been shown to reduce the absorption of oral iron.

Zinc

Zinc compounds induce metallothionein production in intestinal mucosa. This protein binds copper preferentially within duodenal enterocytes and copper absorption into the circulation is thereby reduced. When the enterocyte is shed, metallothionein-bound copper is lost the intestinal lumen. Total body copper falls since copper excretion continues while absorption is reduced. Zinc therapy may act also by inducing hepatocyte metallothionein with concomitant sequestration of intracellular copper, reducing its toxic effects. Guidelines recommend 50 mg of elemental zinc (zinc acetate was the salt studied) three times a day is effective in managing copper overload, but unlike the chelating agents zinc alone is not accepted as treatment for all clinical scenarios (see below).

Food interferes with the absorption of zinc, and it is recommended that zinc be taken 30 minutes before meals.

Zinc salts may affect the absorption of a range of medications (e.g., iron, tetracyclines, fluoroquinolones), and zinc absorption may be reduced by tetracyclines, phosphorus containing compound and iron and calcium suppliments.

If combination treatment with a copper chelator is chosen, there should be at least a one-hour interval between administration of chelator and and zinc (as discussed under the chelators).

Clinical effectiveness

Broadly, the chelators described above, along with zinc salts, may be clinically effective in treating copper overload.

However, Wilson's disease presents in a wide range of ways. Presentation can be from childhood, though adolescence into adulthood. Earlier presentation is usually associated with hepatic disease, fulminant liver failure, or hepatitis (acute or chronic). The neuropsychiatric presentation is seen later during adolescence and early adult life. Patients presenting later may have features of both neurologic and hepatic disease. Presymptomatic individuals may be diagnosed, usually through screening of siblings of affected individuals.

Wilson's disease is rare (approximately 1 in 30 000 births) and this is the primary reason for the lack of randomized controlled trials of treatment regimens. Thus therapeutic recommendations are broadly based on historical data on the outcome of various treatments, together with knowledge of the mode, speed of action of agents and adverse effects. Tetrathiomolybdate remains an investigational drug, and is not commercially available.

In acute fulminant liver failure (coagulopathy and encephalopathy within 8 weeks of the onset of disease) the patient should be referred to a liver transplant centre, as medical therapy is ineffective and emergent liver transplantation is necessary. Outcomes have been published describing a 70–80% one-year survival after transplant. Any patient with a less acute presentation or decompensation of chronic liver disease despite treatment should also be considered for transplantation since treatment with chelators cannot always be relied upon for improvement.

For discussion on the choice of treatment for a patient with Wilson's disease, the reader is referred to the published guidelines. As already noted, clinicians with experience in managing patients with this condition have different opinions and preferences on treatment. In choosing treatment a range of factors need to be remembered, which can make the choice complex, and account for guidelines giving leeway in choice of agents. These include:

- the more severe side effect profile of penicillamine;
- the fact that neurological deterioration may occur after initiation of treatment and that such deterioration may persist;
- the fact that guidelines suggest that introduction of treatment should be gradual – not full dose from the start;
- the issue of noncompliance with treatment in some patients;
- the accepted parameters and targets for monitoring therapy/compliance.

Therefore, access to advice from a clinician experienced in the treatment of Wilson's disease is important, particularly in those with complex clinical disease or without clinical improvement with treatment.

There are also a wide range of agents used generally in patients with Wilson's (pyridoxine, vitamin E, etc.) and more specific agents used to ameliorate neurological features. A diet low in copper rich foods is also recommended in current guidelines.

Adverse effect
Penicillamine

Adverse effects are seen in 10–30% of patients. They may be severe enough to necessitate withdrawal of treatment.

Early (weeks 1–3) side effects include sensitivity reactions with rash, fever, lymphadenopathy, proteinuria, neutropenia and thrombocytopenia. Penicillamine should be stopped if there are early immune side effects. Although in the past reintroduction of penicillamine with steroids was used to try to overcome such effects, the availability of trientine as an effective alternative has made switching therapy the preferred course of action.

Regular monitoring for bone marrow suppression and proteinuria are necessary weekly for the first six to eight weeks and less frequently after this period if no effect is seen.

In patients with neurological features at presentation, initial neurological deterioration has been reported in 10–50% of patients in some studies, and in some cases this deterioration does not reverse.

Late adverse effects of penicillamine (months to years) include nephrotoxicity, a lupus-like syndrome (haematuria, proteinuria, positive antinuclear antibody), bone marrow suppression (aplasia, thrombocytopenia), myasthenia gravis, polymyositis, and loss of taste.

With long-term administration, penicillamine may be associated with several dermatological changes including elastosis perforans serpiginosa and aphthous stomatitis. Progeriatric changes are reported to develop with doses of greater than 1000 mg/day – a reason for reducing to a maintenenace dose as soon as appropriate.

The effects of therapy on pyridoxine metabolism have been discussed earlier.

Trientine

Trientine has fewer reported side effects than penicillamine. Pancytopenia occurs rarely. Renal and hypersensitivity reactions have not been reported. There are case reports of gastrointestinal events. Sideroblastic anaemia and hepatic siderosis may occur if copper deficiency develops with long-term treatment with trientine. Neurological deterioration after starting trientine does occur but the frequency is less studied than with penicillamine.

Zinc

Dyspepsia occurs in some patients, and appears to be least with the acetate salts; this may be ameliorated by using different formulations (e.g., gluconate or sulphate) or altering the time of administration. As with all forms of treatment, copper deficiency can occur. Monitoring of serum copper, non-caeruloplasmin bound copper and 24- hour urine copper will indicate this.

Pregnancy

Although there are concerns with tetratogenicity with penicillamine and trientine, guidelines agree that the risk of stopping treatment during pregnancy outweighs these potential obstetric complications. Since the highest risk of teratogenicity is in the first trimester, lowering the dose of pencillamine at this time has been recommended. In order to reduce the effects of chelators on wound healing and insufficient copper supply to the foetus, some recommend a reduction in dosage in the last trimester. Zinc does not appear to be deleterious to the foetus. Clearly close monitoring of patients with Wilson's disease during pregnancy is necessary and treatment adjusted appropriately. Ideally, copper status is optimized prior to the patient becoming pregnant.

Breastfeeding has not been recommended for patients on chelation therapy, although a report has not found this to be problematic.

Children

Caveats with regard to starting treatment as described above should be observed in children. In guidelines the dose of penicillamine in children is 20 mg/kg/day rounded off to the nearest 250 mg, in two to three divided doses. Although the weight-based dose for trientine has not been established, the same dose as for penicillamine is recommended currently. For zinc salts, in children weighing less than 50 kg, a daily dosage of 75 mg elemental zinc per day is recommended, given in three divided doses.

Table 11.4 shows the pregnancy categories for the agents referred to in this chapter. Table 11.5 summarizes the key points of the agents.

Table 11.4 Pregnancy category (according to United States FDA Pharmaceutical Pregnancy Categories)	
Medication	Category
Ursodeoxycholic acid	B
Penicillamine	D
Trientine	C
Zinc	A

Table 11.5 Key points

Therapy	Mode of action	Pros	Cons	Notes
Ursodeoxycholic acid	Suppresses hepatic synthesis and secretion of cholesterol. Inhibits intestinal absorption of cholesterol. Protection against cytotoxicity of hydrophobic bile acids Choleretic Protection of hepatocytes against apoptosis	Dissolves gallstones in selected patients Value in early PBC	Other treatments preferred except rarely Value in PSC questioned High dose associated with increased risk of death and transplantation	Other treatment options preferred
Penicillamine	Copper chelator – urinary excretion of copper	Long experience – successful in majority of patients	Frequency of side effects: -Immunological -Neutropenia -Proteinuria -Neurological deterioration	Efficacious in all patients groups. Some specialists use as first choice despite frequency of side effects
Trientine	Copper chelator – urinary excretion of copper	Less experience than with penicillamine – but data suggest effective as first line treatment Fewer side effects than with penicillamine	Neurological deterioration may occur; frequency uncertain Storage necessary in refrigerator (2–8 °C)	Increasingly accepted as potential first line therapy
Zinc salts	Induce metallothionein – reduce copper absorption	Few side effects Extent of experience mainly in asymptomatic patients	Slower speed of action Gastric intolerance in some patients	Most used in for pre/a-symptomatic patients, and for maintenance therapy. Not recommended for treatment phase of hepatic presentation

Recommended reading

Ala A, Walker AP, Ashkan K *et al.* (2007) *Lancet* **369**: 397–408.

Askari FK, Greenson, Dick RD *et al.* (2003) Treatment of Wilson's disease with zinc. XVIII. Initial treatment of the hepatic decompensation presentation with trientine and zinc. *J Lab Clin Med* **142**: 385–90.

Bacq Y, Sentilhes L, Reyes HB *et al.* (2012) Efficacy of ursodeoxycholic acid in treating intrahepatic cholestasis of pregnancy. A meta analysis. *Gastroenterology* **143**: 1492–1501.

This meta analysis contains the best evidence for the benefit of UCDA, greatly reducing pruritus in the mother and improving fetal outcomes.

Brewer GJ (2000) Recognition, diagnosis and management of Wilson's disease. *PSEBM* **223**: 39–46.

Brewer GJ, Dick RD, Johnson VD, *et al.* (1998) Treatment of Wilson's disease with zinc: XV: Long-term follow up studies. *J Lab Clin Med* **132**: 264–78.

Brewer GJ, Johnson VD, Dick RD, *et al.* (2000) Treatment of Wilson's disease with zinc. XVII: treatment during pregnancy. *Hepatology* **31**: 364–70.

Brewer GJ, Askari F, Lorincz MT, *et al.* (2006) Treatment of Wilson Disease with ammonium tetrathiomolybdate. IV. Comparison of tetrathiomolybdate and trientine in a double-blind study of treatment of the neurologic presentation of Wilson disease. *Arch Neurol* **63**: 521–7.

A comparative study of trientine and tetrathiomolybdate (TTM; an investigational drug), presenting data which support further study of TTM as a treatment option in Wilson's disease.

Chappell LC, Gurung V, Seed PT, *et al.* (2012) Ursodeoxycholic acid versus placebo, and early term delivery versus expectant management, in women with intrahepatic cholestasis of pregnancy: semifactorial randomized clinical trial. *BMJ* 344:e3799.

Corpechot C, Abenavoli L, Rabahi N, *et al.* (2008) Biochemical response to ursodeoxycholic acid and long term prognosis in primary biliary cirrhosis. *Hepatology* **48**: 871–7.

This is an observational study which demonstrates amelioration of liver function tests with UCDA in biochemical responders which resulted in improvement in long-term outcomes. As there was no UCDA group, it is possible that UCDA may be a means to select those with a slow natural history of the disease.

Czlonkowska A, Gajda J, Rodo M (1996) Effects of long-term treatment in Wilson's disease with D-penicillamine and zinc sulphate. *J Neurol* **243**(3): 269–7.

EASL (2012) Clinical practice guidelines: Wilson's disease. *J Hepatol* **56**: 671–85.

This is the most recent set of guidelines for the diagnosis and management of Wilson's disease written by an international panel of experts.

Ferenci P (2005) Wilson's disease. In: B Bacon, JG O'Grady, A DiBisceglie, JR Lake (eds), *Comprehensive Clinical Hepatology*. Maryland Heights, MS: Elsevier Mosby, Chapter 24, pp. 351–67.

A comprehensive review of Wilson's disease with cumulative data collated from several published sources including useful data on treatment and issues in pregnancy.

Goulis J, Leandro G, Burroughs AK (1999) Randomised trials of ursodeoxycholic acid in primary biliary cirrhosis: a meta-analysis. *Lancet* **354**: 1053–60.

The first meta-analysis, later confirmed by a Cochrane group, that showed that in RCTs with a wide spectrum of severity of PBC, UDCA therapy did not influence long-term outcomes.

Gong Y, Huang ZB, Christensen E, *et al*. (2008) Ursodeoxycholic acid for primary biliary cirrhosis. *Cochrane Database of Systematic Reviews* **3**: CD00051. doi.10.1002/14651858,PMID 18677775.

Joint Formulary Committee (2013) Interactions with penicillamine. *British National Formulary (BNF)* **65**: 914.

Lindor KD, Kowdley KV, Luketic VA, *et al*. (2009) High dose ursodeoxycholic acid for the treatment of primary sclerosing cholangitis. *Hepatology* **50**: 804–14.
UDCA given as 28–30 mg/Kg in PSC is associated with an increase hazard of earlier death compared to placebo, despite statistically significant amelioration in liver function tests. Whether the detrimental effect of this high dose of UDCA applies to other cholestatic diseases remains to be determined.

May GR, Sutherland LR, Shaffer EA (1993) Efficacy of bile acid therapy for gallstones dissolution: a meta-analysis of randomized trials. *Aliment Pharmacol Ther* **7**: 139–48.
Good evidence for the benefit of UDCA for gall bladder stone dissolution in selected patients.

Messner U, Gunter HH, Niesert S (1998) Wilson's disease and pregnancy. Review of the literature and case report. *Z Geburtshilfe Neonatol* **202**: 77–9.

Omata M, Yoshida H, *et al*. (2007) A large scale multicenter double blind trial of ursodeoxycholic acid in patients with chronic hepatitis C. *Gut* **56**: 1747–53.
Evidence that UCDA ameliorates liver function tests in noncholestastic disease without affecting clinical outcome.

Paediatric Formulary Committee (2008) Ursodeoxycholic acid. In: *British National Formulary for Children*. Pharmaceutical Press, London, p. 91.

Paumgartner G, Beuers U (2002) Ursodeoxycholic acid in cholestatic liver disease: mechanisms of action and therapeutic use revisited. *Hepatology* **36**: 525–31.

Poupon R (2012) Ursodeoxycholic acid and bile-acid mimetics as therapeutic agents for cholestatic liver diseases: an overview of their mechanisms of action. *Clinics and Research in Hepatology and Gastroenterology* **36**: S3–S12.

Roberts EA, Schilsky ML (2008) AASLD practice guidelines: diagnosis and treatment of Wilson's disease: an update. *Hepatology* **47**: 2089–2111.

Scheinberg IH, Sternlieb I (1975) Pregnancy in penicillamine-treated patients with Wilson's disease. *N Engl J Med* **293**: 1300–2.

Schilsky ML (2013) Treatment of Wilson's disease. www.uptodate.com (last updated 24 July 2013; last accessed September 2013)
This is the most up-to-date review on the treatment of Wilson's disease, and is a resource that is regularly updated.

Schilsky ML, Scheinberg IH, Sternlieb I (1994) Liver transplantation for Wilson's disease: indications and outcome. *Hepatology* **19**(3): 583–7.

Uy MC, Talingdan-Te MC, Espinosa WZ, *et al*. (2008) Ursodeoxycholic acid in the prevention of gallstone formation after bariatric surgery: a meta-analysis. *Obes Surg* **18**: 1532–38.
Best evidence for the pre emptive use of UCDA to prevent gall stone formation in patients subjected to bariatric surgery.

Walshe JM (2009) The conquest of Wilson's disease. *Brain* **132**: 2289–95.

Weiss KH, Gotthardt D, Klemm D, *et al.* (2011) Zinc monotherapy is not as effective as chelating agents in treatment of Wilson disease. Gastroenterology 2011;140:1189-98.

Weiss KH, Thurik F, Gotthardt DN, *et al.* (2013) Efficacy and safety of oral chelators in treatment of patients with Wilson disease. *Clin Gastroenterol Hepatol* Mar. 28. piiS1542-3565. Epub ahead of print.

Comparative analysis of the outcome of treatment with penicillamine and trientine in a large cohort of patients.

Wilson SAK (1912) Progressive lenticular degeneration: a familial nervous disease associated with cirrhosis of the liver. *Brain* 34: 295–507.

CHAPTER 12

Agents for the treatment of portal hypertension

Karen L. Krok[1] and Andrés Cárdenas[2]

[1]Penn State Milton S. Hershey Medical Center, Hershey, PA, USA
[2]University of Barcelona, Hospital Clinic, Barcelona, Spain

Introduction

Patients with end stage liver disease will suffer from portal hypertension and the complications associated with portal hypertension. These include variceal bleeding, ascites, hepatorenal syndrome, hyponatremia, and hepatic encephalopathy.

Portal pressure is the product of portal blood inflow and resistance to flow. Portal pressure increases initially secondary to an increased resistance to flow through the scarred-down, cirrhotic liver. In addition, there is an increase in portal venous inflow secondary to the splanchnic arteriolar vasodilatation. Portal hypertension then leads to the formation of porto-systemic collaterals. A hepatic venous pressure gradient (HVPG) of > 10 mmHg will result in the formation of varices, and these will bleed at pressures > 12 mmHg. Pharmacologic agents are selected with the goal to decrease the HVPG to <12 mmHg or 20% from baseline. These include nonselective beta-blockers (propranolol, nadolol, and carvedilol), nitrates, vasopression analogs and somatostatin analogs.

Hepatorenal syndrome (HRS) is a condition in which there is progressive kidney failure in a person with cirrhosis. It is a serious and often life-threatening complication of cirrhosis. Several pharmacological agents have been studied to treat HRS. The best available therapy is the use of vasoconstrictors (terlipressin, midodrine, noradrenaline) along with albumin. The most studied vasoconstrictor is terlipressin. Results from randomized controlled studies and systematic reviews indicate that treatment with terlipressin together with albumin is associated with a response rate of approximately 40–50%. However, terlipressin is not yet available in some countries, including the United States. If terlipressin is

Pocket Guide to Gastrointestinal Drugs, Edited by M. Michael Wolfe and Robert C. Lowe. © 2014 John Wiley & Sons, Ltd. Published 2014 by John Wiley & Sons, Ltd.

not available, most centers use "triple therapy," that is octreotide given subcutaneously, albumin and midodrine.

Ascites is the most common complication of cirrhosis that leads to hospital admission. Once ascites develops, mortality is 15% in 1 year and 44% in 5 years. The hallmark of the treatment of ascites is the use of oral diuretics and salt restriction. The usual diuretic regimen consists of an oral dose of furosemide and spironolactone. Single-agent spironolactone is recommended for the first episode of ascites, but given its long half-life and the risk of hyperkalemia, it is often combined with furosemide. Furosemide is not used as a single agent in these patients, and most patients will require dual therapy.

Hypervolemic or dilutional hyponatremia, defined as a serum sodium < 130meq/L, is usually seen in patients with cirrhosis and ascites. It is seldom morbid unless it is rapidly corrected. It is estimated that 22% of patients with advanced cirrhosis have serum sodium levels < 130 mEq/L; however, in patients with refractory ascites or HRS, this proportion may increase to more than 50%. First-line treatment of hyponatremia is free water restriction and discontinuation of diuretics. If these do not work, one could consider an aquaretic medication such as tolvaptan.

Hepatic encephalopathy is the occurrence of confusion, altered level of consciousness and/or coma as a result of liver disease. It is caused by the accumulation in the bloodstream of toxic substances that are normally removed by the liver. It is generally precipitated by an infection, medication noncompliance, gastrointestinal bleeding, dehydration, electrolyte disturbance, shunt placement, or the use of medications that suppress the central nervous system (i.e., narcotics or benzodiazepines). Treatment of hepatic encephalopathy relies on suppressing the production of the toxic substances in the intestine and is generally done with the laxative lactulose or with nonabsorbable antibiotics.

This chapter will focus on drug therapies for patients with complications of portal hypertension.

Nonselective beta-blockers (NSBB)

Mechanism of action/pharmacology

Propranolol and nadolol are nonselective beta-blockers that block both β_1 and β_2 receptors competitively. In the treatment of portal hypertension, they act principally on β_2 receptors, resulting in splanchnic vasoconstriction and a reduction in portal inflow. Carvedilol is a nonselective beta blocker as well as an α_1 blocker. It is proposed that in addition to its β_2 effects causing splanchnic vasoconstriction, it also has an additional effect by reducing intrahepatic portal resistance. For this reason, it is a more potent reducer of the HVPG than propranolol and nadolol.

NSBBs are almost completely absorbed following oral administration. Much of the administered drug is metabolized by the liver during its first passage through the portal circulation. However, somewhat less of the drug is removed during the first circulation through the liver after repeated administration, which accounts for a gradual increase in half-life of the drug after chronic oral administration.

Clinical effectiveness

NSBBs are recommended for both primary prophylaxis and secondary prophylaxis of variceal bleeding. Patients who have survived a variceal bleed, should be treated with NSBBs and endoscopic band ligation to prevent rebleeding (secondary prophylaxis). Primary prophylaxis should be offered to patients with medium to large varices and those patients with small varices that are Childs B/C class or have red wale marks on their varices. Patients without varices should not be prescribed a NSBB, as a large multicenter placebo-controlled double-blind trial failed to show any benefit in the prevention of varix formation in patients with cirrhosis and portal hypertension but no varices at the time of enrollment. Dosages of specific agents are listed in Table 12.1.

Toxicity

Although relatively well tolerated, there are some side effects of NSBBs that need to be mentioned. There will be a reduction in heart rate and blood pressure; the goal in treating patients is to maintain a heart rate of 55–60 beats per minute. If heart rate is continually <50 beats per minute and/or the systolic blood pressure is < 85 mm Hg then the NSBB should be discontinued. There also is a possible increase in airway resistance, making the presence of asthma or chronic obstructive pulmonary disease a contraindication to the use of a NSBB. These agents also augment the hypoglycemic action of insulin and so patients who are susceptible for hypoglycemia should be educated about the warning signs of hypoglycemia.

NSBBs have been assigned a pregnancy class C by the Food and Drug Administration (FDA). These agents can lead to intrauterine growth retardation, neonatal hypoglycemia, hypotension and bradycardia. Only a small amount is expressed in breast milk if the patient is considering breastfeeding.

It should be noted that there is the potential for deleterious effects in patients with refractory ascites. In one single center study, 151 patients with refractory ascites were studied; 51% of patients were treated with NSBB. The median survival was 20 months in patients without a NSBB and only 5 months in patients receiving a NSBB. These authors have proposed that NSBB are contraindicated in patients with refractory ascites.

Table 12.1 Medications used in the treatment of variceal prevention and bleeding

Medication	Class	Dosage	Pregnancy class	Major side effects
Propranolol (Inderal, Inderal LA)	NSBB	**Short acting:** start at 20 mg twice a day and titrate to HR of 60 bpm **Long acting:** start at 80 mg/day and titrate to HR of 60 bpm **Max dose:** 320 mg	C	Hypotension, hypoglycemia, fatigue, shortness of breath, impotence, peripheral circulation dysfunction
Nadolol (Corgard)	NSBB	Start at 20 mg daily and titrate to HR of 60 bpm. **Max dose:** 240 mg	C	
Carvedilol (Coreg)	NSBB	Start at 6.125 mg twice a day and titrate to HR of 60 bpm **Max dose:** 12.5 mg twice a day	C	
Isosorbide mononitrate	Nitrate	Start at 10 mg daily **Max dose:** 40 mg twice a day	C	Headache, hypotension, dizziness
Terlipressin	Vasopressin Analogue	2 mg every 4 hours intravenously; titrate down to 1 mg every 4 hours once there is control of hemorrhage	Not assigned yet as not available in USA	Vasoconstriction and ischemic complications; abdominal pain; arrhythmias; skin necrosis; hyponatremia
Octreotide	Somatostatin Analogue	Bolus of 50 mcg followed by 50 mcg/hour for up to 5 days	B	Rare and minor: Nausea, Vomiting, Abdominal pain, Diarrhea

Nitrates

Mechanism of action/pharmacology

Isosorbide mononitrate (ISMN) is an organic nitrate and is a potent venodilator. Venodilators theoretically act by decreasing intrahepatic and/or portocollateral resistance. There is also a systemic hypotensive effect and the decrease in portal pressure may be more related to a decrease in flow secondary to the systemic hypotension rather than a decrease in resistance. ISMN has excellent bioavailability following oral administration.

Clinical effectiveness

NSBB are first line in the treatment of varices but nitrates can be used if there is a contraindication to a NSBB. Dosage of ISMN is listed in Table 12.1.

Toxicity

Postural hypotension may develop in patients; this effect is accentuated by the presence of alcohol and a NSBB. It is for this reason, that it is uncommon to combine NSBB and ISMN in patients despite data showing a decrease in rates of rebleeding from esophageal varices in patients taking combination therapy. ISMN has been assigned a pregnancy class C by the FDA.

Vasopressin analogs

Terlipressin is a potent vasopressin analog. Although currently not available in the United States, it is used routinely in other parts of the world.

Mechanism of action/pharmacology

Vasopressin is the most potent splanchnic vasoconstrictor. It reduces blood flow to all splanchnic organs, thereby leading to a decrease in portal venous inflow and subsequently to a decrease in portal pressure. Unfortunately, the clinical utility of vasopressin is limited by its potent vasoconstrictive properties which lead to its multiple side effects – cardiac and peripheral ischemia, arrhythmias, hypertension and bowel ischemia. For this reason, terlipressin, a synthetic vasopressin analog, has been utilized. It has a longer biological activity and significantly fewer side effects than vasopressin. Terlipressin acts on V_1 receptors to cause splanchnic vasoconstriction, which reduces portal inflow and hence portal pressures.

Clinical effectiveness

Although not yet available in the United States, it is used elsewhere in the world as first-line treatment for hepatorenal syndrome (HRS) and variceal bleeding. A meta-analysis of studies of terlipressin demonstrated a 52% efficacy in reversing HRS. For variceal bleeding, the initial dose is 2 mg every 4 hours intravenously and then titrated down to 1 mg every 4 hours once there is control of hemorrhage. After three days, terlipressin should be discontinued. The dose is different, though, for HRS. It is dosed at 1 mg every 4–6 hours and then increasing it to 2 mg every 4 hours. The dose is titrated to aim for a 10% increase in mean arterial pressure and/or reduction in creatinine to a level below 1.5 mg/dL.

Toxicity

There are several adverse events that are associated with terlipressin; however, these occur in less than 10% of patients. These are mostly related to vasoconstriction and ischemic complications. Regular examination of the skin, limb peripheries, and cardiovascular system should be done while a patient is on therapy. The initial dose is 2 mg every 4 hours intravenously and then titrated down to 1 mg every 4 hours once there is control of hemorrhage. V_2 receptor blockade by terlipressin results in free water absorption in the renal collecting ducts leading to a dilutional hyponatremia; this resolves rapidly upon discontinuation of the medication.

As it is not available in the United States, it has not been assigned a pregnancy class by the FDA yet. In Australia, though, it was given a pregnancy class D. Dosages are listed in Table 12.1.

Somatostatin analog

The most commonly used somatostatin analog is octreotide.

Mechanism of action/pharmacology

Somatostatin analogs cause splanchnic vasoconstriction at pharmacological doses. Their exact mechanism of action is unclear.

Clinical effectiveness

The benefit of octreotide is that it can be used for 5 days or longer. However, results of meta-analyses show that there is a negligible benefit with the use of octreotide as a single agent. The reason that octreotide alone may not be beneficial is that it is associated with tachyphylaxis.

A continuous infusion is required as its actions on hepatic and systemic hemodynamics are transient. Dosages for variceal bleeding are listed in Table 12.1. In the treatment of HRS, it is given subcutaneously 100 mcg three times a day with an increase to 200 ug t.i.d. if needed. Octreotide alone is ineffective. Dosages for HRS are noted in Table 12.2.

Table 12.2 Medications used in the treatment of hepatorenal syndrome

Medication	Class	Dosage	Pregnancy class	Major side effects
Octreotide	Somatostatin Analogue	100 mcg subcutaneously three times a day **Max dose:** 200 mcg three times a day	B	Rare and minor: nausea, vomiting, abdominal pain, diarrhea
Midodrine	Antihypertensive	5 mg three times a day **Max dose:** 12.5 mg three times a day	C	Headache, rash, flushing, dry mouth, anxiety, confusion
Albumin	Volume expander	50–100 gm/day	N/A	Rare
Terlipressin	Vasopressin Analogue	0.5–1 mg every 4–6 hours and increasing it to 2 mg every 4 hours. Titrate to an aim for a 10% increase in mean arterial pressure and/ or reduction in creatinine below 1.5 mg/dL	Not assigned yet as not available in USA	Vasoconstriction and ischemic complications; abdominal pain; arrhythmias; skin necrosis; hyponatremia

Toxicity

Octreotide has relatively fewer side effects than terlipressin and is relatively well tolerated. It has been assigned a pregnancy class B by the FDA.

Midodrine

Mechanism of action/pharmacology

Midodrine is a vasopressor/antihypotensive agent. Midodrine is a α_1-receptor agonist and exerts its actions via activation of the *alpha-adrenergic receptors* of the arteriolar and venous vasculature, producing an increase in vascular tone and elevation of blood pressure. The recommended dose of midodrine is 7.5 mg orally three times a day with an increase to 12.5 mg three times a day if needed. Midodrine is rapidly absorbed after an oral dose.

Clinical effectiveness

Midodrine is used in combination with octreotide and albumin in the treatment of HRS. There are only case series demonstrating the benefit of this regimen, although hepatologists routinely prescribe this when a diagnosis of HRS is made.

Toxicity

Midodrine should not be used in patients with persistent hypertension, pheochromocytoma or thyrotoxicosis. It is well tolerated and has some minor side effects, which include headache, flushing face, confusion, dry mouth, nervousness, anxiety and rash. The FDA has assigned it a pregnancy class C. Specific dosages are listed in Table 12.2.

Albumin

Mechanism of action/pharmacology

Albumin is a sterile preparation of 5 or 25% serum albumin obtained by fractioning blood from human donors. The 25% solution is routinely used in the treatment of HRS. Typically a patient receives 1gm/kg as first dose and the 20–40 gm of 25% solution daily in combination with either terlipressin or octreotide and midodrine.

Clinical effectiveness

Albumin is used in combination with either octreotide and midodrine or terlipressin in the treatment of HRS. It should be noted that in the clinical trials evaluating the effectiveness of terlipressin, the arm without albumin did not respond as well. This implies that albumin plays a crucial role in the treatment of HRS. It is also used to diagnose HRS – if a patient does not respond to 2 days of albumin infusion then a diagnosis of HRS is more likely than simply a pre-renal condition.

Toxicity

Albumin is well-tolerated. As it is a blood product, it is safe during pregnancy.

Loop diuretics

Mechanism of action/pharmacology

Loop diuretics act by inhibiting the luminal Na-K-2Cl symporter in the thick ascending limb of the loop of Henle in the kidney. This results in a reduction in the reabsorption of sodium chloride, hence promoting a diuresis. The most commonly used loop diuretic is furosemide. The bioavailability of furosemide is about 65% after an oral dose.

Clinical effectiveness

Loop diuretics are part of the standard of care in the treatment of ascites and volume overload. The doses of oral diuretics (loop diuretics and aldosterone antagonists) can be increased simultaneously every 5 days, maintaining the ratio of spironolactone 100 mg to furosemide 40 mg. The maximum dose is 400 mg of spironolactone and 160 mg of furosemide. This ratio usually maintains normokalemia. The goal is to induce a weight loss of 0.5 kg/day if no edema is present and 1.0 kg/day in patients with peripheral edema.

Toxicity

There are many side effects that can occur with the use of loop diuretics. As with many diuretics they can lead to dehydration and electrolyte imbalance (including potassium, calcium, sodium and magnesium). Aggressive use can also lead to a metabolic alkalosis. Hyperuricemia also is relatively common. The FDA has given this a pregnancy class C. The dosage of furosemide is listed in Table 12.3.

Table 12.3 Medications used in the treatment of ascites

Medication	Class	Dosage	Pregnancy class	Major side effects
Furosemide (Lasix)	Loop diuretic	Start at 20–40 mg/day and increase every 3–5 days **Max dose:** 160 mg/day	C	Dehydration, electrolyte imbalance, hyperuricemia
Spironolactone (Aldactone)	Aldosterone antagonist	Start at 50–100 mg/day and increase every 3–5 days **Max dose:** 400 mg/day	C	Hyperkalemia, gynecomastia, minor GI side effects

Aldosterone antagonist

Mechanism of action/pharmacology
Aldosterone antagonists are competitive antagonists of the actions of mineralocorticoids, of which aldosterone is the most potent naturally occurring compound. They bind to the aldoscterone receptor and prevent it from assuming the active conformation. These receptors are present in the late distal tubule and collecting system in the nephron. The overall action of aldosterone is to enhance sodium reabsorption and potassium secretion; hence by blocking aldosterone activity, diuresis can occur.

Clinical effectiveness
Aldosterone antagonists are standard of care in the treatment of ascites and volume overload. The doses of both oral diuretics (loop diuretics and aldosterone antagonists) can be increased simultaneously every 5 days, trying to maintain the ratio of spironolactone 100 mg to furosemide 40 mg.

Toxicity
About 70% of an oral dose of spironolactone is absorbed. The most serious toxic effects of spironolactone result from hyperkalemia. In addition, painful gynecomastia and minor gastrointestinal symptoms can occur. It has been given a pregnancy class C by the FDA. The dosage of spironolactone is listed in Table 12.3.

Aquaretics

Mechanism of action/pharmacology
Tolvaptan is a selective, competitive vasopressin receptor (V2) antagonist that promotes aquaresis. It blocks arginine vasopressin from binding to V2 receptors in the distal nephron and this induces the excretion of electrolyte-free water without changing the total level of electrolyte excretion. By doing this it allows for an improvement in serum sodium.

Clinical effectiveness
The approval of tolvaptan for the treatment of hyponatremia is based on two randomized controlled trials examining the use of tolvaptan versus placebo in the treatment of hyponatremia. There is little data on its use in patients also using diuretics. Hyponatremia recurs after withdrawal of the tolvaptan.

Toxicity
There are a few side effects that have been reported in clinical trials. These include dry mouth, thirst and dehydration. The adverse event that

Table 12.4 Medication used in treatment of hyponatremia

Medication	Class	Dosage	Pregnancy class	Major side effects
Tolvaptan (Samsca)	Aquaretic	15 mg/day and increase if serum sodium is <136 mmol/L and had increased by <5 mmol/L **Max dose:** 60 mg/day	C	Dry mouth, thirst, hypernatremia

is most feared is a rapid rise in serum sodium. There is also small risk in gastrointestinal bleeding perhaps related to the effect of tolvaptan on vitamin K dependent clotting factors and platelets. And more recently there was evidence of elevated liver enzymes in patients receiving tolvaptan to treat polycystic kidney disease at doses of 90 mg/day (which is higher than the 60 mg/day maximum dose that is recommended in patients with hyponatremia). It was given a pregnancy class C by the FDA. Table 12.4 lists dosing details.

Disaccharides

Mechanism of action/pharmacology

Lactulose is a disaccharide that is not absorbed by the digestive tract. It is thought to reduce the generation of ammonia by bacteria, render ammonia unabsorbable by converting it to ammonium (NH_4), and increase transit of bowel content through the gut. By doing so, it prevents and treats hepatic encephalopathy.

Clinical effectiveness

There are few clinical trials examining the use of lactulose in patients with encephalopathy, but clinical experience has shown repeatedly that lactulose is effective in this patient population. It would be unethical to do a placebo-controlled trial with lactulose given the clinical experience showing improvement with lactulose. Patients are instructed to titrate this medication for a goal of 2–4 soft bowel movements/day. This typically requires 15–30 ml three times a day.

Toxicity

Patients often struggle with lactulose as it has a very sweet taste; it is recommended to take this with fruit juice to mask the taste. In addition,

Table 12.5 Medications used for the treatment of hepatic encephalopathy

Medications	Class	Dosage	Pregnancy class	Major side effects
Lactulose	Disaccharide	15–30 mL 3–4 times a day and titrate to 3–5 bowel movements/day	B	Diarrhea, dehydration, bloating
Rifaximin (Xifaxan)	Non-absorbable antibiotic	550 mg twice a day or 400 mg three times a day	C	Rare and minor; Nausea, vomiting, abdominal pain, rash

lactulose leads to significant (and at times unpredictable) diarrhea and so patients feel limited in their ability to perform their daily activities. Bloating can also occur. The FDA has classified lactulose as pregnancy class B. See Table 12.5 for further dosing details.

Antibiotics

The antibiotics neomycin and metronidazole were previously used as treatment for hepatic encephalopathy. Given their many side effects, they were not well tolerated for use long term. There have been a few studies examining rifaximin for the use of treatment of hepatic encephalopathy, but it was a large randomized placebo-controlled trial in 2010 that confirmed the role of rifaximin in the treatment of encephalopathy. This study concluded that patients receiving rifaximin remained free of hepatic encephalopathy more than those in the placebo group and also had a decreased rate of hospitalization. Because of this, rifaximin is now a mainstay of treatment for hepatic encephalopathy and will be the only antibiotic discussed here.

Mechanism of action/pharmacology

Rifaximin is a semisynthetic antibiotic based on rifamycin. It has poor oral bioavailability and hence very little of it is absorbed when taken orally. Rifaximin interferes with *transcription* by binding to the β-subunit of bacterial *RNA polymerase*. This results in the blockage of the translocation step that normally follows the formation of the first phosphodiester bond, which occurs in the transcription process. The rationale for its use is the fact that ammonia and other waste products are generated and converted by intestinal bacteria, and killing of these bacteria would reduce the generation of these waste products.

Clinical effectiveness
In the landmark study described above, rifaximin significantly decreased the risk of a recurrence in hepatic encephalopathy (45.9% in placebo versus 22.1% in the rifaximin treated group).

Toxicity
It is a remarkably well-tolerated medication with very few side effects. The biggest (and often prohibitory) concern is the cost of the medication. Many insurance companies do not pay for this medication and it can cost upwards of $1000/month to pay for this out of pocket. The FDA has assigned it pregnancy class C. See Table 12.5 for further dosing details.

Recommended reading

Abid S, Jafri W, Hamid S, *et al.* (2009) Terlipressin vs. octreotide in bleeding esophageal varices as an adjuvant therapy with endoscopic band ligation: a randomized double-blind placebo-controlled trial. *Am J Gastroenterol* **104**: 617–23.

Angeli P, Volpin R, Gerunda G, *et al.* (1999) Reversal of type 1 hepatorenal syndrome with the administration of midodrine and octreotide. *Hepatology* **29**: 1690–7.
This study has been used as the basis for the "triple therapy" for HRS and it included only 13 patients. It did show an improvement in survival and renal function in patients on octreotide and midodrine compared to dopamine.

Bass NM, Mullen KD, Sanyal A, *et al.* (2010) Rifaximin treatment in hepatic encephalopathy. *N Engl J Med* **362**: 1071–81.
This study compared placebo to rifaximin in patients with a previous history of hepatic encephalopathy. Rifaximin significantly decreased the risk of hospitalization and recurrence of hepatic encephalopathy.

Garcia-Tsao G, Sanyal A, Grace N, *et al.* (2007) Prevention and management of gastroesophageal varices and variceal hemorrhage in cirrhosis. *Hepatology* **46**: 922–38.

Gluud LL, Christensen K, Christensen E, *et al.* (2012) Terlipressin for hepatorenal syndrome. *Cochrane Database Syst Rev* **9**.

Martin-Llahi M, Pepin M, Guevara M, *et al.* (2008) Terlipressin and albumin versus albumin in patients with cirrhosis and hepatorenal syndrome: a randomized study. *Gastroenterology* **134**: 1352–9.
The addition of terlipressin to albumin improved renal function in 43.5% of patients compared to 8.7% in patients with albumin alone. This is a landmark trial.

Runyon B (2009) Management of adult patients with ascites due to cirrhosis: an update. *Hepatology* **49**: 2088–2107.

Schrier RW, Gross P, Gheorghiade M, *et al.* (2006) Tolvaptan, a selective oral vaso-pressin V2-receptor antagonist, for hyponatremia. *N Engl J Med* **355**: 2099–2112. *This study showed a significant increase in serum sodium in patients at day 4 and 20 of tolvaptan use.*

Serste T, Melot C, Francoz C, *et al.* (2015) Deleterious effects of beta-blockers on survival in patients with cirrhosis and refractory ascites. *Hepatology* **52**: 1017–22. *This study examined the use of beta blockers in patients with refractory ascites and found a survival of only 5.0 months in patients on NSBB versus 20.0 months in patients not on NSBB.*

Sidhu SS, Goyal O, Mishra BP, *et al.* (2011) Rifaximin improves psychometric per-formance and health-related quality of life in patients with minimal hepatic encephalopathy (RIME trial). *Am J Gastroenterol* **106**: 307–16.

CHAPTER 13

Pancreatic enzymes

Steven J. Czinn and Samra S. Blanchard
University of Maryland School of Medicine, Baltimore, MD, USA

Introduction

Pancreatic enzyme replacement therapy is currently the standard treatment for nutrient malabsorption secondary to pancreatic insufficiency. This treatment is safe and effective in reducing steatorrhea and fat malabsorption. It is well tolerated and has few side effects. Effective therapy has been limited by the ability to replicate the physiologic process of enzyme delivery to the appropriate site (typically the duodenum) at the appropriate time. The challenges include enzyme destruction in the stomach, lack of adequate mixing with the chyme in the duodenum, and failure to deliver and activate at the appropriate time. The goals of management are to improve absorption of fat, prevent steatorrhea, and improve nutritional status. The use of oral therapy pre-dates the creation of the US Food and Drug Administration (FDA) in 1938, and currently enzyme replacement is the standard therapy in patients diagnosed with malabsorption secondary to pancreatic insufficiency.

The composition and various formulations of pancreatin and pancrelipase affect their use and ability to deliver appropriate amounts of active enzyme to the duodenum. Pancreatin, a crude mixture, is derived from swine or ox pancreas, and each milligram contains no less than 2 United States Pharmacopeia (USP) units of lipase and 25 USP units of amylase and protease activity. Pancrelipase is obtained from swine pancreas and is a more concentrated and purified enzyme preparation. Each milligram contains no less than 24 USP units of lipase and 100 USP units of amylase and protease activity. Because of its higher enzyme content, pancrelipase formulations are favored over pancreatin preparations.

In April 2004, the FDA declared that all orally administered pancreatic enzyme products are considered new drugs and will require the submission and approval of an new drug application (NDA) if manufacturers wished to continue marketing their products.

Pocket Guide to Gastrointestinal Drugs, Edited by M. Michael Wolfe and Robert C. Lowe. © 2014 John Wiley & Sons, Ltd. Published 2014 by John Wiley & Sons, Ltd.

An understanding of the labeling of the enzyme preparations is important in order to administer the correct dosages. Preparations in the United States are demarcated by the amount of lipase contained in 1 pill and are dosed in USP units. The USP unit for lipase administration is roughly 3 times the value of international units (IU), which are used in academic publications.

Mechanism of action

The exocrine pancreas is responsible for synthesis and secretion of digestive enzymes including lipase, co-lipase, phospholipase, protease, and amylase, into the duodenum in an alkaline, bicarbonate-rich fluid. In exocrine pancreatic insufficiency, the pancreolipase products contain lipase, protease and amylase. These enzymes catalyze the hydrolysis of fats into monoglycerides, free fatty acids and glycerol, proteins into peptides and amino acids and starches into alpha-dextrins which are then digested by gluco-amylase to maltose and maltriose.

Because lipase is the most sensitive enzyme to proteolytic degradation in acidic environment, fat malabsorption occurs sooner than protein deficiency and is usually the more clinically relevant nutritional problem. Inactivation of pancreatic enzymes occur when pH levels drop below 4.0. The need for protection from proteolytic degradation and gastric acid inactivation has led the development of enteric coated formulations that have been shown to increase absorption compared to uncoated preparations. The uncoated formulations are currently used largely in clinical practice to treat the pain of chronic pancreatitis but not the malabsorption.

Enteric-coated preparations were designed to avoid inactivation in the stomach, as the enzyme is protected from the acidic environment by the coating, and dissolves in the duodenum when pH exceeds 5 to 5.5.

During a meal, normal pancreatic secretion delivers more than 360 000 IU (>1 million USP units) of active lipase into the duodenum in healthy adults, of which 10% is needed to prevent fat malabsorption.

Dosing and schedule of administration

All pancreatic enzyme replacement therapy drugs approved in United States are reviewed in Table 13.1. All pancreatic enzyme supplements are enteric coated except Viokace, which therefore must be taken with proton pump inhibitors. Pertzye has additional bicarbonate buffering compared to other enteric coated products. Available doses of FDA approved products are also summarized in Table 13.1. Currently there is no generic pancreatic enzyme supplement available in the United States.

Table 13.1 Pancreatic enzymes – brand names available in USA

	Lipase units	Amylase units	Protease units
Pancreolipase™	5000	27 000	17 000
Creon®			
Creon 3 000	3 000	15 000	9500
Creon 6 000	6 000	30 000	19 000
Creon 12 000	12 000	60 000	38 000
Creon 24 000	24 000	120 000	76 000
Ultresa™			
Ultresa 13 800UL	13 800	27 600	27 600
Ultresa 20 700UL	20 700	41 400	41 400
Ultresa 23 000UL	23 000	46 000	46 000
Zenpep®			
Zenpep 3 000	3 000	16 000	10 000
Zenpep 5 000	5 000	27 000	17 000
Zenpep 10 000	10 000	55 000	34 000
Zenpep 15 000	15 000	82 000	51 000
Zenpep 20 000	20 000	109 000	68 000
Zenpep 25 000	25 000	136 000	85 000
Pancreaze™			
Pancreaze MT4	4 200	17 500	10 000
Pancreaze MT10	10 500	43 750	10 000
Pancreaze MT16	16 800	70 000	40 000
Pancreaze MT20	21 000	61 000	37 000
Pertzye™			
Pertzye	8 000	30 250	28 750
Pertzye	16 000	60 500	57 500
Viokace®			
Viokace	10 440	39 150	39 150
Viokace	20 880	78 300	78 300

Dosing is adjusted based on the amount of lipase in the supplements. The initial dose aims to supply 40–60 IU/minute of lipase activity within the duodenal lumen. To achieve this goal in adults, approximately 25 000 to 40 000 IU of lipase is required to digest a typical meal, and about 5000 to 25 000 IU of lipase per snack.

Dosage recommendations for pancreatic enzyme replacement therapy were published following the Cystic Fibrosis Foundation Consensus Conferences. It was found that lipid digestion was better when enzymes were taken during or after meals. The capsule may also be opened and the contents can be added to a small amount of acidic food such as applesauce. The contents of the capsule should not be chewed or crushed. This is especially important in treatment of infants. The ingredients of the capsule cannot be mixed with infant formula or breast milk, and should be given in applesauce prior to feeding. Infants need 2000–4000 lipase units of enzyme per 120 ml of breast milk or infant formula.

For patients who cannot tolerate oral feedings, Creon® pancrelipase pellets can be mixed with any baby food with a pH less than 4.5 and administered via large diameter gastrostomy tubes (14 French or larger) without clogging, sticking or visible pellet damage, and with no loss of gastric resistance or lipase activity.

Enzyme dosing should begin with 1000 lipase units/kg of body weight per meal for children less than age 4 years to a maximum of 2500 lipase units/kg of body weight per meal (or less than or equal to 10 000 lipase units/kg of body weight per day), or less than 4000 lipase units/g fat ingested per day.

For children 4 years of age and older, the enzyme dosing should begin with 500 lipase units/kg of body weight per meal to a maximum of 2500 lipase units/kg of body weight per meal (or less than or equal to 10 000 lipase units/kg of body weight per day), or less than 4000 lipase units/g fat ingested per day.

Enzyme doses expressed as lipase units/kg of body weight per meal should be decreased in older patients because they weigh more but tend to ingest less fat per kilogram of body weight.

Dosing should be adjusted based on body weight, clinical symptoms and stool fat content. Changes in dosage may require an adjustment period of several days. If doses are to exceed 2500 lipase units/kg of body weight per meal, further investigation is warranted. Doses greater than 2500 lipase units/kg of body weight per meal (or greater than 10 000 lipase units/kg of body weight per day) should be used with caution and only if they are documented to be effective by 3-day fecal fat measures that indicate a significantly improved coefficient of fat absorption. Doses greater than 6000 lipase units/kg of body weight per meal have been associated with colonic stricture, indicative of fibrosing colonopathy, in children less than 12 years of age.

Monitoring therapy

Currently there are no guidelines in clinical practice for monitoring the efficacy of enzyme replacement therapy and determining a need for dose adjustment. In research studies, a commonly used method to monitor therapy is the use of the coefficient of fecal fat absorption (CFA). The CFA uses a 72-hour stool collection comparing the amount of lipid ingested with that excreted. The cumbersome nature of stool studies limits their use in the outpatient setting. Commonly, the efficacy of therapy is determined by clinically assessing the patient's weight, height and BMI, assessing exocrine pancreatic insufficiency-related GI signs and symptoms, and following blood levels of important micronutrients and fat soluble vitamins.

Adverse effects

The most commonly reported side effects for recently approved enzymes are headache (6%), dizziness (6%), abdominal pain (9%), and flatulence. Historically, hyperuricemia, and hyperuricosuria, which leads to dysuria and uric acid crystaluria, have been reported in cystic fibrosis patients using older formulations. Porcine-derived pancreatic enzyme products contain purines that may increase blood uric acid levels.

Allergic reactions may occur and caution should be exercised when administering pancrelipase to a patient with a known allergy to proteins of porcine origin.

Potential irritation of oral mucosa can occur if the pancreatic enzymes are crushed or chewed or mixed in foods having a pH greater than 4.5. These actions can disrupt the protective enteric coating resulting in early release of enzymes, irritation of oral mucosa, and/or loss or enzyme activity.

The most concerning adverse effect associated with enzyme replacement is fibrosing colonopathy, which has been described in cystic fibrosis patients receiving more than 24 000 IU of lipase/kg daily. This is characterized by submucosal collagen deposition with fibrosis and varying degrees of stricturing. Some studies suggest that the acid-resistant coating of enzyme preparations may be responsible for the fibrosing colonopathy, as it has also been demonstrated with other medications that use the same methacrylic copolymer coating. In addition, as these cases largely occurred with high-dose enzyme therapy (>50 000 IU/kg daily), limits are suggested for maximum dosage and delivery. Caution should be used when doses exceed 2500 IU/kg per meal or 10 000 units per kilogram per day.

All pancreatic enzyme supplements are Pregnancy Category C. The risk and benefit of pancrelipase should be considered in the context of the need to provide adequate nutritional support to a pregnant woman with exocrine pancreatic insufficiency. Adequate caloric intake during pregnancy is important for normal maternal weight gain and fetal growth. Reduced maternal weight gain and malnutrition can be associated with adverse pregnancy outcomes.

It is not known whether this drug is excreted in human milk, and caution should be exercised when pancreatic enzyme therapy is administered to a nursing woman. The risk and benefit of pancrelipase should be considered in the context of the need to provide adequate nutritional support to a nursing mother with exocrine pancreatic insufficiency.

Recommended reading

Borowitz DS, Grand RJ, Durie PR, *et al.* (1995) Use of pancreatic enzyme supplements for patients with cystic fibrosis in the context of fibrosing colonopathy. *Journal of Pediatrics* **127**: 681–4.

Borowitz DS, Baker RD, Stallings V (2002) Consensus report on nutrition for pediatric patients with cystic fibrosis. *Journal of Pediatric Gastroenterology Nutrition* Sep; **35**: 246–59.

Creon package insert (2011) North Chicago, IL: Abbott Laboratories.

Fieker A, Philpott J, Armand M (2011) Enzyme replacement therapy for pancreatic insufficiency: present and future. *Clinical and Experimental Gastroenterology* **4**: 55–73.

FitzSimmons SC, Burkhart GA, Borowitz D, *et al.* (1997) High-dose pancreatic-enzyme supplements and fibrosing colonopathy in children with cystic fibrosis. *N Engl J Med* **336**(18): 1283–9.
  This is a review of patients who developed fibrosing colonopathy during pancreatic enzyme treatment.

Pancreaze package insert (2011) Titusville, NJ: Janssen Pharmaceuticals, Inc.

Pertzye package insert (2012) Bethlehem, PA Digestive Care.

Shlieout G, Koerner A, Maffert M, *et al.* (2011) Administration of CREON® Pancrelipase pellets via gastrostomy tube is feasible with no loss of gastric resistance or lipase activity: an *in vitro* study. *Clin Drug Investig* **31**(7): e1–7.
  This is a study to demonstrate effective drug administration via large bore gastrostomy tube.

Stallings VA, Start LJ, Robinson KA, *et al.* (2008) Evidence-based practice recommendations for nutrition-related management of children and adults with cystic fibrosis and pancreatic insufficiency: results of a systematic review. *Journal of the American Dietetic Association* **108**: 832–9.

Ultresa package insert (2012) Aptalis Pharma US, Inc., Birmingham, AL.

Viokace package insert (2012) Birmingham, AL Aptalis Pharma US.

Zenpep package insert (2011) Yardley, PA: Eurand Pharmaceuticals, Inc.

ANTIMICROBIALS AND VACCINES

PART IV

CHAPTER 14

Antibiotics for the therapy of gastrointestinal diseases

Melissa Osborn

MetroHealth Medical Center, Case Western Reserve University, Cleveland, OH, USA

Introduction

Antimicrobials are used to treat a wide variety of gastrointestinal infections, including infectious diarrhea, *Clostridium difficile* colitis, *Helicobacter pylori* and intra-abdominal infections, such as cholecystitis, diverticulitis, appendicitis and abscess. Virtually every class of antimicrobial can be used for some type of infection related to the gastrointestinal system. In this chapter, the most commonly used antimicrobials to treat these infections will be discussed (Table 14.1). The choice of antibiotic depends upon whether the causative agent is known (as with *C. difficile* or *H. pylori*) or whether treatment is empiric (as in diverticulitis or cholecystitis). Antivirals for viral hepatitis and antiparasitics for helminths will not be discussed.

Pharmacologic properties

Beta-lactams

The beta-lactams include the penicillins and the cephalosporins. They share a similar ring structure, with side chains determining antibacterial spectrum and pharmacologic properties. Both classes work by inhibiting cell wall synthesis via binding to penicillin-binding proteins (PBPs). Resistance to beta-lactams is conferred by bacterial enzymes that hydrolyze the beta-lactam ring (beta-lactamases), which can be overcome by the addition of a beta-lactamase inhibitor to the penicillin. All beta-lactams are considered bactericidal.

The bioavailability of the penicillins and cephalosporins vary widely, but oral absorption is moderate at best. The most commonly used beta-lactams for gastrointestinal infections are amoxicillin, piperacillin-tazobactam,

Pocket Guide to Gastrointestinal Drugs, Edited by M. Michael Wolfe and Robert C. Lowe. © 2014 John Wiley & Sons, Ltd. Published 2014 by John Wiley & Sons, Ltd.

Table 14.1 Antimicrobials for the treatment of gastrointestinal infections

Generic name	Brand names	Adult dosing	Pediatric dosing	Pregnancy class
Amoxicillin	Amoxil, Clamoxyl, Doxamil, Hiconcil, Polymox, Trimox	500 mg PO TID 1 g PO BID (triple therapy) or TID (dual therapy) for *H pylori*	40 mg/kg/day divided q8 hours	B
Piperacillin-tazobactam	Zosyn,Tazocin	3.375 g IV q6 hours 3.375 g IV q4 hours (for *Pseudomonas* coverage)	100 mg/kg IV q6 hours	B
Ampicillin-sulbactam	Unasyn, Bacimex, Combactam	1.5–3 g IV q6 hours	100–300 mg/kg IV divided q6 hours	B
Ticarcillin-clavulanate	Timentin	3.1 g IV q6 hours	75 mg/kg IV q6 hours	B
Cefoxitin	Mefoxitin	1–2 g IV q6–8 hours	80–160 mg/kg divided q6 hours	B
Ceftriaxone	Rocephin, Rocephalin, Rocephine	1–2 g IV q24 hours	50 mg/kg IV q24 hours	B
Ceftazidime	Ceptaz, Foram, Fortaz, Fortum, Kefadim, Tazicef, Tazidime	1–2 g IV q8–12 hours	50 mg/kg IV q8 hours	B
Imipenem	Primaxin, Tienam	500 mg IV q6 hours	15–25 mg/kg IV q6 hours (max 4 g/day)	C
Meropenem	Merrem, Meronem	1 g IV q8 hours	60–120 mg/kg q8 divided q8 hours	B

Drug	Brand names	Adult dose	Pediatric dose	Category
Ertapenem	Invanz	1g IV q24 hours	15 mg/kg IV q12 hours (max 1 g/day)	B
Doripenem	Doribax	500 mg IV q8 hours	Not established	B
Ciprofloxacin	Cipro, Cifox, Ciloxan, Ciproxin,	400 mg IV q12h 500–750 mg PO q12h	Not recommended due to cartilage toxicity	C
Levofloxacin	Levaquin, Cravit, Quixin, Tavanic	500–750 mg IV q24h 500–750 mg PO q24h		C
Moxifloxacin	Avelox, Vigamox	400 mg IV/PO q24h		C
Tigeglycline	Tygacil	100 mg IV × 1 then 50 mg IV q12h	Not established; use under age 8 not recommended	D
Metronidazole	Flagyl, Elyzol, Protostat, Rozex	500 mg IV/PO q8–12 hours	7.5 mg/kg IV/PO q6 hours	B
Vancomycin	Vancocin, Lyphocin, Vancoled, Vancor	125 mg PO QID	40 mg/kg in 3 or 4 divided doses (max 2 grams)	C
Rifaximin	Xifaxan, Lumenax	Traveler's diarrhea: 400 mg PO BID × 3 d Hepatic encephalopathy: 550 mg PO BID	No recommendations for children <12 years old	C
Fidaxomicin	Dificid	200 mg PO BID	Not studied	B
Azithromycin	Zithromax, Azitromax, Sumamed, Zitromax, Z-Pak, Tri-Pak, ZMax	500 mg PO daily	10 mg/kg IV/po q24 hours	B
Clarithromycin	Biaxin, Biclar, Klacid, Zeclar	500 mg PO BID	7.5 mg/kg PO q12 hours (max 1 g/day)	B

ampicillin-sulbactam, ticarcillin-clavulanic acid, cefoxitin, ceftriaxone, and ceftazidime. All except amoxicillin are only available intravenously. With the exception of ceftriaxone, all are metabolized by the kidney and thus require dosage adjustment in kidney disease. Ceftriaxone is excreted largely through the biliary system. Both penicillins and cephalosporins are highly protein bound, and they therefore do not penetrate well intracellularly. The distribution into most tissues, however, is adequate. The most important toxicities with the beta-lactams are hypersensitivity reactions, including anaphylaxis, rash, and allergic interstitial nephritis. Cross-reactivity between penicillin allergy and cephalosporin allergy is variable and depends on the nature of the penicillin allergy, as well as the similarity between the side chain of the penicillin causing the reaction and the cephalosporin to be used.

Carbapenems

There are four carbapenems approved for clinical use: imipenem, meropenem, ertapenem, and doripenem. Like the beta-lactams, the carbapenems inhibit bacterial cell wall synthesis by binding to penicillin binding proteins. They are not well-absorbed orally and must therefore be administered intravenously. All are metabolized by the kidney and require dose-adjustment in the presence of renal insufficiency. Drug interactions are minimal, although levels of valproic acid can be lowered by carbapenems. Adverse effects are primarily related to hypersensitivity. All of the carbapenems (imipenem in particular) lower the seizure threshold and have been associated with seizures in clinical use. Importantly, ertapenem does not provide coverage against *Pseudomonas aeruginosa*, so its use should be avoided in infections where this pathogen is suspected. All other carbapenems possess good coverage against *Pseudomonas*.

Fluoroquinolones

The fluoroquinolones are synthetic antimicrobials, with each successive generation of agents having a different antimicrobial spectrum. The most widely used fluoroquinolones are the second-generation agents ciprofloxacin and levofloxacin and the fourth generation agent moxifloxacin. Ciprofloxacin and levofloxacin have gram-negative coverage (including susceptible *Pseudomonas*), with levofloxacin having more gram-positive coverage than ciprofloxacin. Moxifloxacin offers broad spectrum coverage against gram-positive, gram-negative and anaerobic organisms, but not *Pseudomonas*.

All of the fluoroquinolones act by inhibiting two bacterial enzymes, DNA gyrase and topoisomerase IV. Through inhibition of these enzymes, bacterial cell replication is impaired, followed rapidly by cell death. They are well absorbed and penetrate into tissues well, with levels in some tissues exceeding serum levels. The bioavailability of ciprofloxacin is ~70–80%, and even higher for levofloxacin (99%) and moxifloxacin (90%). Therefore, oral therapy is nearly equivalent to parenteral therapy in persons with an intact small bowel. Once absorbed, ciprofloxacin and levofloxacin are metabolized by the kidney (and require dose adjustment in renal disease), while moxifloxacin is metabolized by the hepatic and biliary systems.

Drug interactions are minimal with fluoroquinolones, which do not affect the cytochrome P450 system, with the exception of the CYP1A2 enzyme (responsible for metabolism of methylxanthines, caffeine, methadone, clozapine). Co-adminstration of warfarin with a fluoroquinolone can result in prolongation of the prothrombin time. Absorption of the oral fluoroquinolones is also decreased by co-administration of divalent cations, such as aluminum, calcium, iron and magnesium. Therefore, antacids and dietary supplements (as well as milk and milk-containing products) should be discontinued or avoided near the dosing interval of the fluoroquinolone to prevent suboptimal serum levels of the drug.

Nausea and diarrhea are the most commonly reported adverse effects of the fluoroquinolones. Rash is infrequent (0.4–2.8%), as is anaphylaxis. Liver enzyme elevations occur in 2–3% and are mild and reversible upon discontinuation of the drug. More serious toxicities include tendinopathy and QT prolongation. Fluoroquinolone-related tendinopathy occurs most often in the Achilles tendon and can occur anywhere from 2 hours to 6 months after the first dose. Rupture of the tendon occurs in up to 50% of cases. Risk factors for tendinopathy include kidney disease, dialysis and renal transplant. Prolongation of the QT interval is also a class effect and can lead to *torsades de pointes* in patients at risk. Ciprofloxacin has a lower risk of QT prolongation with consequent *torsades de pointes* than levofloxacin or moxifloxacin. Risk factors for fluoroquinolone-associated torsades include co-administration with another QT-prolonging drug (particularly class III or class IA antiarrhythmics), underlying cardiac disease, renal impairment, hypokalemia or hypomagnesemia, and female sex.

The utility of the fluoroquinolones for the treatment of gastrointestinal infections has been hindered by growing widespread resistance to these agents, particularly among *Escherichia coli* and *Camplylobacter jejuni*. The decision to use a fluoroquinolone to treat a gastrointestinal infection should be guided by knowledge of local resistance patterns in the area of acquisition (i.e., in cases of traveler's diarrhea) and by the results of antimicrobial susceptibility testing when available.

Glycylcyclines

Tigecycline is a bacteriostatic agent related to the tetracycline class. It binds to the 30S ribosomal subunit and blocks entry of transfer RNA into the ribosome. The peptide chain cannot elongate, and protein synthesis is inhibited. It is available only intravenously. The volume of distribution is large, indicating extensive distribution into tissues, with highest levels in bone and bone marrow. Most of the drug is excreted unchanged by the biliary system, with smaller portions undergoing glucuronidation by the liver, and <30% excreted unchanged in the urine. No dosage adjustments are required in renal insufficiency. No dosage adjustments are recommended in mild hepatic impairment (Child A or B cirrhosis), but in Child C cirrhosis, the maintenance dose is reduced to 25 mg IV every 12 hours. Caution should be used in this population. There are no major drug interactions with tigecycline.

The most common adverse effects of tigecycline are nausea and vomiting, which occur in up to 30% of patients. These symptoms can be dose-limiting and can be lessened by administering anti-emetics or food at the time of infusion. Symptoms usually begin in the first 1–2 days of treatment and are more common in younger patients and women.

Tigecycline has broad spectrum coverage of gram-positive, gram-negative and anaerobic organisms. It retains activity against methicillin-resistant *S aureus* and vancomycin-resistant enterococci. It has no *Pseudomonas* activity, but is active against some strains of resistant *Acinetobacter*.

Glycopeptides

Vancomycin is a glycopeptide that works through inhibition of cell wall synthesis in dividing bacteria. Although it is most commonly used in its intravenous form for serious gram-positive infections such as methicillin-resistant *S. aureus*, its most common use in gastrointestinal infections is in its oral form for *C. difficile*. Intravenous vancomycin concentrates poorly in the stool and is ineffective in treating *C. difficile*.

When given orally or per rectum, vancomycin is poorly absorbed from the gastrointestinal tract, even when pseudomembranous colitis is present. It is excreted unchanged in the feces. Because of the lack of systemic absorption, drug interactions are not significant with oral administration. Adverse effects are also minimal, and oral vancomycin is well-tolerated. There is a risk of selection for vancomycin-resistant enterococci with use of oral vancomycin, but the incidence and clinical significance of this risk has not been firmly established.

Macrolides

The macrolide antibiotic class contains the agents erythromycin, clarithromycin, and azithromycin. Because of their improved gastrointestinal tolerability and less frequent dosing, the latter two agents have largely replaced erythromycin in clinical use. All drugs in this class are bacteriostatic, and exert their effect by inhibiting bacterial protein synthesis via binding to the bacterial 50S ribosomal subunit. The oral bioavailability of clarithromycin (~50%) is greater than that of azithromycin (37%), but both drugs are widely distributed in tissues. Clarithromycin is metabolized primarily by the liver, with about 20% excreted unchanged in the urine. Metabolites are also excreted in the urine. Renal insufficiency increases the half-life of clarithromycin, and doses should be adjusted for a creatinine clearance less than 30 milliliters per minute. Azithromycin is mainly excreted unmetabolized through the feces via biliary excretion, although a small portion is also metabolized through demethylation. No dosage adjustments are necessary with renal or hepatic failure.

There are no important drug interactions with azithromycin. Clarithromycin, however, interacts with the cytochrome P450 CYP 3A system and can affect levels of drugs metabolized by this group of enzymes (Table 14.2) The absorption of azithromycin is impeded

Table 14.2 Selected drug interactions between antimicrobials and other agents

Antimicrobial	Interacting agents
Carbapenems (imipenem, doripenem, meropenem, ertapenem)	Valproic acid
Azithromycin	Cyclosporine, digoxin, nelfinavir, pimozide
Clarithromycin	Carbamazepine, cimetidine, cisapride, **colchicine**, cyclosporine, digoxin, disopyramide, disulfiram, dofetilide, ergot alkaloids, lidocaine, loratadine, lovastatin, midazolam, phenytoin, pimozide, repaglinide, rifampin, rifabutin, ritonavir, saquinavir, simvastatin, sildenafil, tacrolimus, terfenadine, theophylline, valproic acid, verapamil, warfarin, zidovudine
Fluoroquinolones	**Antacids** (with magnesium, aluminum, calcium, or zinc), **amiodarone**, cyclosporine, didanosine, **iron**, methadone, nitrofurantoin, NSAIDs, oral contraceptives, oral hypoglycemics, phenytoin, **procainamide**, rasagiline, rifampin, rifabutin, sucralfate, tizanidine, theophylline, warfarin
Metronidazole, Tinidazole	Alcohol, azathioprine, cimetidine, cyclosporine, disulfiram, fluorouracil, lithium, warfarin, phenobarbital, For tinidazole: phenytoin, drugs metabolized by CYP 3A4

by administration with food, or magnesium- or aluminum- containing antacids, and the dose should be separated in time from either of these. The most common adverse effects of both macrolides are nausea, vomiting and diarrhea. Rare, but more serious adverse events, are cholestatic hepatitis with azithromycin and ventricular tachycardias and acute psychosis with clarithromycin. Less serious elevations of liver enzymes can also be seen which are reversible with cessation of the drug.

Nitroimidazoles

The most commonly used nitroimidazole is metronidazole. A second generation nitroimidazole, tinidazole, is also available for the treatment of giardiasis, amebiasis, and vaginal infections. Metronidazole exerts its action via production of free radicals that are toxic to the bacterium. Once the drug enters the cell, it becomes activated by reduction of its nitro group, which accepts electrons from host electron transport proteins. A concentration gradient forms, and metronidazole radicals lead to breakage and destabilization of microbial nucleic acids.

Oral doses of metronidazole are almost completely absorbed, for nearly 100% oral bioavailability. Penetration into tissues is good, including the central nervous system, biliary tree, brain abscesses, liver abscesses, and peritoneal fluid. It is metabolized via oxidation of its side chains by the hepatic CYP P450 system before being excreted primarily in the urine, and to a lesser extent in the feces. Because of its dependence on this CYP P450 system for metabolism, there have been reports of drug interactions between metronidazole and other drugs affecting CYP 3A4, such as amiodarone, carbamazepine, cyclosporine, phenobarbital, tacrolimus and warfarin.

The most common adverse effects with metronidazole are gastrointestinal, including nausea and anorexia. Pancreatitis and hepatitis have been described. Many people report dysgeusia while taking metronidazole. Persons taking metronidazole should avoid alcohol while on therapy, as concomitant use of this drug with alcohol can cause a disulfiram-like reaction characterized by tachycardia, hypotension, flushing and palpitations.

The antimicrobial spectrum of metronidazole includes most ananerobes, including gram-positives and gram-negatives, and certain parasitic diseases (*Entamoeba histolytica, Trichomonas vaginalis, Giardia lamblia*). It is the first-line agent for the treatment of *C. difficile*. Resistance to metronidazole among strict anaerobes is rare, but there has been increasing resistance seen among isolates of *Giardia* and *H. pylori*. Some countries report *H. pylori* resistance rates as high as 70%.

Rifaximin

Rifaximin is a nonabsorbable semisynthetic derivative of rifamycin. It is approved for uncomplicated traveler's diarrhea and for the treatment of hepatic encephalopathy. It inhibits the beta subunit of the bacterial DNA-dependent RNA polymerase, leading to a disruption in RNA synthesis via chain termination. It remains in the intestinal lumen, with a bioavailability of <0.4%. Most of the drug is excreted unchanged in the feces. Because the drug is not absorbed, there are no drug interactions, and few drug adverse effects. Compared to placebo, rifaximin has no additional toxicities or safety considerations.

Rifaximin should not be used for cases of traveler's diarrhea where invasive mucosal disease or systemic infection is suspected due to its nonabsorbability. It is also not recommended for dysentery due to *Shigella*, *Campyobacter* or *Salmonella*.

Fidaxomicin

Fidaxomicin is a novel macrocyclic antibiotic approved for the treatment of *C. difficile* infection. It is bactericidal and inhibits nucleic acid synthesis by impairing initiation of RNA synthesis and inhibiting the RNA polymerase. The drug is not absorbed well orally, and the poor systemic bioavailability leads to high levels in the colon at the site of action. Because it is not absorbed, drug interactions are not significant. The most common adverse effects reported with fidaxomicin are nausea, vomiting, anemia, and neutropenia. Compared to other treatments for *C. difficile*, fidaxomicin is thought to have less effect on the normal flora, with specific activity against *C. difficile* and relatively poor activity against enteric bacteria and anaerobic gram-negatives that constitute the normal colonic flora. Isolates of the epidemic strain of *C. difficile* BI/NAP1/027 tend to require higher minimal inhibitory concentrations to fidaxomicin than non-epidemic strains, which does not, however, seem to significantly affect its efficacy.

Clinical uses

Infectious diarrhea

The differential diagnosis for infectious diarrhea takes into consideration the patient's immune status, travel history, sick contacts, local epidemiology (such as ongoing outbreaks), and acuity of illness. As dictated by the clinical scenario, diagnostic testing for bacterial pathogens includes culture for *Salmonella*, *Shigella* and *Campylobacter*, and testing for *C. difficile* toxin. Special testing is required for isolation of *E. coli* O157: H7. In severe cases of diarrhea, empiric therapy with a fluoroquinolone (ciprofloxacin 500 mg orally twice daily or levofloxacin 500 mg orally daily for 3–4 days) is appropriate if there is a high clinical suspicion for a community-acquired enteric pathogen, pending identification and susceptibility testing. If there has also been recent antibiotic exposure, additional empiric coverage with metronidazole pending testing for *C. difficile* may also be warranted. Therapy can be modified on the basis of diagnostic results and susceptibility testing.

In cases of traveler's diarrhea, empiric therapy should be driven by the area of acquisition. Rifaximin (200 mg orally three times daily for 3 days) can be used in cases of suspected noninvasive *E. coli* (which causes about 50–75% of traveler's diarrhea in Latin America and Africa), but should be avoided in *Shigella, Salmonella,* or *Campylobacter*. Fluoroquinolones (ciprofloxacin 500 mg orally twice daily for 1–3 days or levofloxacin 500 mg orally daily for 1–3 days) are a better option for these pathogens. Increasing resistance to the fluoroquinolones has been seen, especially among *Campylobacter* in Southeast Asia and Thailand, where azithromycin (1 g PO once or 500 mg orally daily for 3 days) should be considered as an alternative.

In immunocompromised patients, or when diarrhea is persistent beyond 7 days, protozoal pathogens must be considered. The most common is *Giardia,* which can be treated with a course of metronidazole (250 mg orally three times daily for 5 days) or tinidazole (2 grams as a single dose). Other considerations in this scenario include *Cyclospora cayetanensis, Cryptosporidium parvum, Entamoeba histolytica, Isospora belli,* microsporidium, and mycobacteria.

Clostridium difficile

The treatment strategy for an initial episode of *C. difficile* depends on the severity of disease, which is based upon the peripheral white blood cell count, serum creatinine, and presence of shock, ileus or megacolon (Figure 14.1). Mild or moderate cases are treated with metronidazole 500 mg three times per day for 10–14 days. Oral vancomycin (125 mg orally four times per day) is reserved for severe initial episodes. In cases of colitis complicated by hypotension/shock, ileus or megacolon, oral or nasogastric vancomycin plus intravenous metronidazole 500 mg IV every 8 hours is appropriate. First recurrences of *C. difficile* are treated the same way as an initial episode. Second recurrences are managed with a vancomycin taper; after a full 10–14 day course, vancomycin is reduced to 125 mg twice per day for a week, 125 mg once daily for a week, and then 125 mg every 2 or 3 days for 2–8 weeks. A small study of 8 patients found a high cure rate when rifaximin 400 mg twice daily for 14 days was given after the last full course of vancomycin.

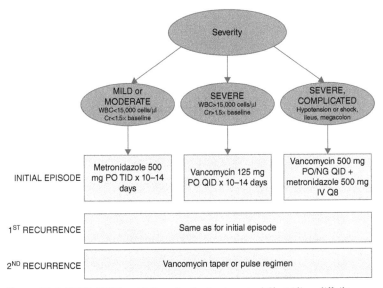

Figure 14.1 SHEA/IDSA guidelines for the treatment of *Clostridium difficile* infection.

The role of fidaxomicin in the treatment of *C. difficile* has not been well-established. In a phase 3 randomized double-blind trial, clinical cure rates for fidaxomicin were noninferior to oral vancomycin. Recurrence rates were lower with fidaxomicin than with vancomycin among non-epidemic strains of *C. difficile*, but were similar with the NAP1/BI/027 strain. The study excluded patients with life-threatening or fulminant *C. difficile* infection, toxic megacolon, or more than one occurrence of *C. difficile* infection within 3 months before the start of the study.

Helicobacter pylori

Eradication of *H. pylori* is achieved with combinations of proton pump inhibitors, bismuth preparations, and antimicrobials. Several regimens have been studied, but growing resistance (especially to clarithromycin) has led to increasing failure rates with some combinations. The optimal initial regimen has not been defined. Table 14.3 lists possible treatment combinations. Regardless of the treatment regimen chosen, a test of cure should be performed in patients with persistent symptoms, those who have had a gastric ulcer or gastric MALT lymphoma, those with a prior ulcer complication or who have

Table 14.3 Regimens for the treatment of *Helicobacter pylori*

Regimen	Agents	Eradication rate	Comments
Triple therapy (7–14 days)	Proton-pump inhibitor* Amoxicillin 1 g twice daily Clarithromycin 500 mg twice daily	<80%	Failure rates high due to clarithromycin resistance
Quadruple therapy (10–14 days)	Bismuth subsalicylate 2 tabs (524 mg) four times per day Tetracycline 500 mg four times per day Metronidazole 500 mg three times per day Omeprazole 20 mg twice a day, or other proton pump inhibitor*	93%	Preferred in areas where the prevalence of clarithromycin resistance is high (>20%) or in patients with repeated exposure to clarithromycin or metronidazole
Sequential therapy	Day 1–5: Proton-pump inhibitor* Amoxicillin 1 g twice daily Day 6–10 Proton-pump inhibitor* Clarithromycin 500 mg twice daily Tinidazole 500 mg twice daily	>90%	

*Rabeprazole 20 mg twice daily, esomeprazole 20 mg twice daily, lansoprazole 30 mg twice daily, pantoprazole 40 mg twice daily.

had gastrectomy for gastric cancer. In addition to consideration of resistant H. pylori, adherence to the treatment regimen should be assessed.

Intra-abdominal infections

The choice of empiric regimen for the treatment of intra-abdominal infections is based upon the severity of presentation and whether the infection is community-onset or hospital-acquired. (Table 14.4) The recommended agents are designed to cover the most likely pathogens in each scenario. For community-acquired infections, treatment should be aimed at enteric gram-negative aerobic and facultative bacilli and enteric gram-positive streptococci. If there is perforation of the distal small bowel, appendix, or colon, coverage for obligate anaerobes should also be provided. Coverage for *Pseudomonas* is generally not important. Single agents or combination regimens may be used. Recently, there have been increasing rates of resistance to ampicillin-sulbactam among *E. coli*. Therefore, ampicillin-sulbactam is no longer recommended in the treatment of intra-abdominal infections. Other single-agent options for treatment for mild-to-moderate infection are cefoxitin, ertapenem, moxifloxacin, tigecycline and ticarcillin-clavulanic acid. For high risk or severe infections, imipenem, meropenem, doripenem or piperacillin-tazobactam should be considered for monotherapy.

Health-care associated infections are more difficult to treat empirically because of the potential for multidrug resistant organisms. Therefore, empiric therapy should be driven by local microbiologic results historically within both the institution and the patient. Multidrug regimens with expanded spectra against gram-negative aerobes and facultative anaerobes are usually needed. The backbone of empiric regimens should include a carbapenem (imipenem, meropenem, doripenem) or a beta-lactam with either a beta-lactamase inhibitor or nitroimidazole (piperacillin-tazobactam or ceftazidime + metronidazole) plus vancomycin if methicillin-resistant *S. aureus* is suspected.

For uncomplicated community-acquired biliary infections, anaerobic therapy is not necessary unless a biliary-enteric anastomosis is suspected. Therapy with a cephalosporin, such as ceftriaxone, is recommended Broader coverage is warranted in severe infections, nosocomial infections, or if the patient is immunocompromised or has advanced age. Choices include the carbapenems, piperacillin-tazobactam, or a fluoroquinolone in combination with metronidazole. Vancomycin should be added if there is a clinical concern for methicillin-resistant *S. aureus*.

Table 14.4 Guidelines for the treatment of intra-abdominal infections in adults from the Infectious Disease Society of America and the Surgical Infection Society

Initial empiric treatment of extra-biliary complicated community-acquired intra-abdominal infection

Regimen	Mild-to-moderate severity: perforated or abscessed appendicitis and other infections of mild-to-moderate severity	High risk or severity: severe physiologic disturbance, advanced age, or immunocompromised
Single agent	cefoxitin 2 g IV q6 hours ertapenem 1 g IV q24 hours moxifloxacin 400 mg IV q24 hours tigecycline 100 mg IV × 1 then 50 mg IV q12 hours ticarcillin-clavulanic acid 3.1 g IV q6 hours	imipenem 500 mg IV q6 hours meropenem 1 g IV q8 hours doripenem 500 mg IV q8 hours piperacillin-tazobactam 3.375 mg IV q6 hours
Combination	cefazolin 1–2 g IV q8 hours OR cefuroxime 1.5 g IV q8 hours OR ceftriaxone 1–2 g IV q24 hours OR cefotaxime 1–2 g IV q6-8 hours OR ciprofloxacin 400 mg IV q12 hours OR levofloxacin 750 mg IV q24 hours OR + metronidazole 500 mg IV q8–12 hours	cefepime 2 g IV q8–12 hours OR ceftazidime 2 g IV q8 hours OR ciprofloxacin 400 mg IV q12 hours OR levofloxacin 750 mg IV q24 hours OR + metronidazole 500 mg IV q8–12 hours

Empiric therapy for healthcare-associated complicated intra-abdominal infection

	Regimen				
Organisms seen at local institution	**Carbapenem**	**Piperacillin-tazobactam**	**Ceftazidime or cefepime, each with metronidazole**	**Aminoglycoside**	**Vancomycin**
<20% resistant *Pseudomonas aeruginosa*, ESBL-producing Enterobacteriaceae, *Acinetobacter*, or other MDR GNB	Recommended	Recommended	Recommended	Not recommended	Not recommended

ESBL-producing Enterobacteriaceae	Recommended	Recommended	Not recommended	Recommended
P aeruginosa >20% resistant to ceftazidime	Recommended	Recommended	Not recommended	Recommended
MRSA	Not recommended	Not recommended	Not recommended	Recommended

Initial empiric treatment of biliary infection in adults

Scenario	Regimen
Community-acquired acute cholecystitis of mild-to-moderate severity	cefazolin 1–2 g IV q8 hours OR cefuroxime 1.5 g IV q8 hours OR ceftriaxone 1–2 g IV q24 hours
Community-acquired acute cholecystitis of severe physiologic disturbance, advanced age, or immunocompromised state; Acute cholangitis following bilio-enteric anastomosis of any severity	imipenem 500 mg IV q6 hours OR meropenem 1 g IV q8 hours OR doripenem 500 mg IV q8 hours OR piperacillin-tazobactam 3.375 mg IV q6 hours
	cefepime 2 g IV q8–12 hours OR ciprofloxacin 400 mg IV q12 hours OR levofloxacin 750 mg IV q24 hours + metronidazole 500 mg IV q8–12 hours
Health care-associated biliary infection of any severity	As above for severe acute cholecystitis plus addition of vancomycin 15–20 mg/kg IV q8–12 hours

Recommended reading

Adachi JA, DuPont HL (2006) Rifaximin: a novel nonabsorbed rifamycin for gastrointestinal disorders. *Clin Infect Dis* Feb.; **42**(4): 541–7.

Cohen SH, Gerding DN, Johnson S, *et al.* (2010) Clinical practice guidelines for *Clostridium difficile* infection in adults: 2010 update by the society for healthcare epidemiology of America (SHEA) and the infectious diseases society of America (IDSA). *Infect Control Hosp Epidemiol* May; **31**(5): 431–55.
These updated guidelines on the management of Clostridium difficile *outline the treatment of both first episodes and recurrences of this infection in mild and severe cases. Guidance on surveillance, diagnosis, and infection control are also included.*

Gilbert DN, Moellering RC, Eliopoulos GM, Chambers HF, Saag MS (eds) (2012) *The Sanford Guide to Antimicrobial Therapy 2012: 42nd Edition*. Sperryville, VA: Antimicrobial Therapy, Inc. No. 1.
The Sanford Guide is a comprehensive, well-referenced pocket guide to antimicrobial therapy which covers all aspects of antimicrobial use, including pharmacokinetics, spectrum, preferred agent by syndrome and organism, dosing, adverse effects and much more.

Guerrant RL, Van Gilder T, Steiner TS, *et al.* (2001) Practice guidelines for the management of infectious diarrhea. *Clin Infect Dis* Feb.; **32**(3): 331–51.
These guidelines address the epidemiology of acute diarrhea, the yield and cost-effectiveness of stool culture, and recommendations for treatment of specific pathogens. An algorithm for diagnosis is provided. In addition, guidelines for public health management of infectious diarrhea are provided.

Jafri NS, Hornung CA, Howden CW (2008) Meta-analysis: sequential therapy appears superior to standard therapy for *Helicobacter pylori* infection in patients naive to treatment. *Ann Intern Med* June; **148**(12): 923–31.

Khaliq Y, Zhanel GG (2003) Fluoroquinolone-associated tendinopathy: a critical review of the literature. *Clin Infect Dis* June; **36**(11): 1404–10.

Louie TJ, Miller MA, Mullane KM, *et al.* (2011) Fidaxomicin versus vancomycin for *Clostridium difficile* infection. *N Engl J Med* Feb.; **364**(5): 422–31.

Malfertheiner P, Bazzoli F, Delchier JC, *et al.* (2011) Helicobacter pylori eradication with a capsule containing bismuth subcitrate potassium, metronidazole, and tetracycline given with omeprazole versus clarithromycin-based triple therapy: a randomised, open-label, non-inferiority, phase 3 trial. *Lancet* Mar.; **377**(9769): 905–13.

Mandell GL, Bennett JE, Dolin R (eds) (2010) *Principles and Practice of Infectious Diseases*. 7th edn. Philadephia, PA: Churchill Livingstone Elsevier; No. 1.
This comprehensive textbook of infectious diseases is considered the premier reference in the field. Chapters on antibiotics, syndromes and individual pathogens are included. Each antimicrobial class is detailed including mechanism of action, pharamacokinetics, adverse effects and clinical uses.

McColl KE (2010) Clinical practice. Helicobacter pylori infection. *N Engl J Med* Apr.; **362**(17): 1597–1604.

Noskin GA (2005) Tigecycline: a new glycylcycline for treatment of serious infections. *Clin Infect Dis* Sep.; **41** Suppl 5: S303–14.

Owens RC, Jr., Nolin TD (2006) Antimicrobial-associated QT interval prolongation: pointes of interest. *Clin Infect Dis* Dec.; **43**(12): 1603–11.

Paterson DL, Depestel DD (2009) Doripenem. *Clin Infect Dis* July; **49**(2): 291–8.

Pawlowski SW, Warren CA, Guerrant R (2009) Diagnosis and treatment of acute or persistent diarrhea. *Gastroenterology* May; **136**(6): 1874–86.

This review article discusses the pathophysiology of bacterial diarrhea, diagnostic methods, epidemiologic settings for diarrhea, and gives an algorithm for the workup and treatment of acute or persistent diarrhea. Included in the algorithm are community-acquired or traveler's diarrhea, nosocomial diarrhea and persistent diarrhea lasting longer than 7 days.

Pepin J (2008) Vancomycin for the treatment of *Clostridium difficile* infection: for whom is this expensive bullet really magic? *Clin Infect Dis* May; **46**(10): 1493–8.

Solomkin JS, Mazuski JE, Bradley JS, *et al.* (2010) Diagnosis and management of complicated intra-abdominal infection in adults and children: guidelines by the Surgical Infection Society and the Infectious Diseases Society of America. *Clin Infect Dis* Jan.; **50**(2): 133–64.

The updated guidelines on the management of intra-abdominal infections highlight diagnostic evaluations, microbiologic evaluation and timing of antimicrobial therapy. Recommended antimicrobial regimens for cholecystitis, cholangitis, and other intra-abdominal infections, both community-acquired and nosocomial, are discussed.

Venugopal AA, Johnson S (2012) Fidaxomicin: a novel macrocyclic antibiotic approved for treatment of Clostridium difficile infection. *Clin Infect Dis* Feb.; **54**(4): 568–74.

CHAPTER 15

Antimicrobials for parasitic diseases

Joachim Richter

University Hospital for Gastroenterology, Hepatology and Infectious Diseases, Heinrich-Heine-University, Düsseldorf, Germany

5-Nitroimidazoles

Introduction

5-Nitroimidazoles were introduced to medicine in 1960 when metronidazole was used to treat *Trichomonas vaginalis*. These compounds were soon found to possess a wide spectrum against intestinal protozoa and anaerobic bacteria and *Helicobacter pylori*.

Mechanism of action

The mechanism of action of these compounds is still not well understood. Presumably the 5-nitro group of drug leads to the breakage of the helical structure of the DNA of the microorganism.

Pharmacology

5-nitroimidazoles can be administered orally, intravenously, rectally or intravaginally. The bioavailability is complete after oral ingestion. The various derivatives vary in the amount of urinary or biliary elimination of the compound and its metabolites.

Clinical effectiveness

Spectrum of 5′nitroimidazoles

5-nitroimidazoles are effective against infections by *Helicobacter pylori*. and anaerobic bacteria (e.g., *Clostridium difficile*), as well as a large variety of intestinal protozoa among these *Entamoeba histolytica, Giardia intestinalis, Trichomonas spp.* (Table 15.1). Whereas clinically decreased susceptibility of *Entamoeba histolytica* sensu stricto is not a frequent problem provided metronidazole is given at a full dose this is not the case in giardiasis. Due to the lack of commercial interest,

---

Pocket Guide to Gastrointestinal Drugs, Edited by M. Michael Wolfe and Robert C. Lowe. © 2014 John Wiley & Sons, Ltd. Published 2014 by John Wiley & Sons, Ltd.

Table 15.1 Treatment of *Entamoeba histolytica* and *Giardia intestinalis*

Organism	Drug of choice and dose	Alternative
Entamoeba histolytica (*sensu stricto*)		
Intestinal carriage	Paromomycin 25–35 mg/ kg/d in 3 divided doses for 5–10 days	1. Diloxanid furoate 500 mg tid for 10 days or 2. Iodoquinol 650 mg tid for 20 days
Invasive E. histolytica s.s. Colitis, amoeboma, extraintestinal amebiasis, liver abscess	Metronidazole 750 mg, tid PO or in severe cases i.v + Paromomycin 25–35 mg/ kg/d for 10 days in 3 divided doses for 10 days Only liver abscesses close to the pericardium: drainage + optionally: Chloroquine (salt) 250 mg bid for 7–20 days	Tinidazole 800 mg tid for 3–5 days + Diloxanid furoate 500 mg tid for 10 days or + Iodoquinol 650 mg tid for 20 days Paromomycine
Giardia intestinalis	Tinidazole 1 g bid for 2–5 days Ornidazole 500 mg qid for 5 days Secnidazole 1000 mg/d for 3 days Metronidazole *750 mg* tid for 3–5 days	resistant (combined two-drug therapy): add Paromomycin *25–35 mg/ kg/d for 10 days in 3 divided doses for 10 days* or Mebendazole *200 mg tid for 3–5 days* or Albendazole 10–15 mg/ kg/d for 3 days Multiresistant (combined triple therapy): add: chloroquine (salt) 250 mg bid for 7–20 days or nitazoxanide 500 mg/d bid for 3–10 days

controlled studies on the efficacy of 5-nitroimidazole are scarce, but clinicians worldwide report that the susceptibility of *Giardia* is decreasing. Therefore, first and even second therapy attempts with a single drug frequently fail. Unfortunately no systematic study has been undertaken so far to establish a sound algorithm for the therapy of multiresistant giardiasis (Escobedo *et al.*, 2007). Patients who do not clear giardiasis after several treatment attempts should be investigated for immune-suppression e.g., IgA deficiency and HIV infection. Patients with CVID (common variable immune deficiency) are particularly difficult to treat. A tentative algorthithm proposes the use of one 5-nitroimidazole (tinidazole, secnidazole, ornidazole) as first line therapy, and to switch to another 5-nitro-imidazole while adding another substance class (e.g., paromomycine) at the second attempt. If both fail, chloroquine or nitazoxanide may be added and therapy courses extended (Table 15.1)

Toxicity
Side effects of 5-nitroimidazoles if given for less than ten days are usually mild and reversible, and most frequently include nausea, vomiting, metallic taste and intolerance to alcohol. CNS side effects (e.g., dizziness and sleepiness) occur more frequently in metronidazole therapy as compared to the other 5-nitroimidazole derivatives. In long-term high dose therapy leucopenia, agranulocytosis, hallucinations, peripheric polyneuropathy and convulsions have been reported.

All nitroimidazoles are pregnancy category C, not because of embryotoxic and teratogenic effects but of mutagenic and cancerogenic effects with high dose long-term-administration in animals. If possible, 5-nitroimidazoles should not be given during the first trimester. Excretion into breast milk is rapid, and nursing should be suspended during 5-nitroimidazole therapy

Imidazole derivatives with generic and brand names
Metronidazole: Flagyl, Clont
Tinidazole: Fasigyne, Simplotan, Tricolam
Secnidazole: Flagentyl
Ornidazole: Tiberal
Nimorazole: Esclama

Benzimidazoles

Introduction
Benzimidazoles were first developed for veterinary medicine where several compounds are used including albendazole, flubendazole, fenbendazole and triclabendazole. Mebendazole was introduced first into human medicine followed by thiabendazole which, however, was not well tolerated and was replaced in the 1980s by albendazole. Triclabendazole was also widely used in Veterinary Medicine before its introduction in man in the 1990s (Millán *et al.*, 2000; Keiser *et al.*, 2005)

Mechanism of action

All benzimidazoles have a similar mechanism of action on nematodes. These drugs bind to helminth tubules with subsequent inhibition of polymerization to microtubules. Benzimidazoles are usually absorbed several fold if taken with a fatty meal. Albendazole has a more rapid tissue diffusion than mebendazole. Triclabendazole and its active sulfoxide metabolite are primarily excreted in the bile.

Pharmacology

All benzimidazoles are taken orally. Whereas metabolites of mebendazole are inactive, sulfoxide metabolites of albendazole and triclabendazole are highly active.

Clinical effectiveness

Mebendazole is less well absorbed from the intestine than albendazole and undergoes an important first pass effect in the liver with transformation to inactive metabolites. It is inexpensive and particularly useful in intestinal nematode infections, e.g., pinworm, whipworm and hookworm infections (Table 15.2). It has been replaced by albendazole in the treatment of echinococcosis but constitutes an alternative in patients with albendazole hepatitis (Brunetti *et al.*, 2010; Eckert *et al.*, 2011).

Albendazole has a rapid tissue diffusion and a broad spectrum not only against some larval and adult nematodes (hookworms, *Ascaris lumbricoides, Loa loa* filariae) but also against the metacestode stage of human cestodes (Table 15.2). It is the drug of choice for cysticercosis and echinococcosis. Benzimidazoles have some antiprotozoal activity against *G. intestinalis* and the microsporidia *Encephalitozoon spp.* Due to its higher excretion in bile, mebendazole seems to be more effective than albendazole in this respect (Escobedo *et al.* 2007).

Triclabendazole is the drug of choice for trematode infections due to the large liver flukes *Fasciolia hepatica, F. gigantica* and the lung flukes *Paragonimus spp.* In the future, it might play a role in echinococcosis therapy (Richter *et al.*, 2013) (Table 15.2). Triclabendazole is available through the World Health Organization or from the manufacturer (Keiser and Utzinger 2004; Keiser *et al.*, 2005).

Toxicity

The most important adverse events occurred when used for extended periods of time at high doses, as for echinococcosis. These include reversible hepatitis, bone marrow depression and alopecia. Reported side effects of triclabendazole after single- or double-dose administration are due to its efficacy but not to pharmacological toxicity: biliary colic due to the expulsion of liver flukes or parasite fragments through the biliary

Table 15.2 Indications for benzimidazole compounds and ivermectin. Alternative therapies

Organism	Drug of choice and dose	Alternative
Angiostrongylus	*Prednisone* 40–60 mg/kg/d for 3–5 days than tapered + *Albendazole* 7.5 mg/kg bid for 6 days	Helminths die spontaneously within months, sometimes surgery required
Anisakis spp	endoscopic or surgical removal	*Albendazole* 400 mg bid for 3 days
Ascaris lumbricoides	*Mebendazole* 100 mg bid for 3 days	1. *Albendazole* 500 mg once, 2. *Pyrantel* 10 mg base/kg once, 3. *Piperazine* 75 mg/kg once for 2–4 days, 4. *Levamisole.* 150 mg once
Capillaria philippinensis	*Albendazole* 200 mg bid for 10 days	*Mebendazole* 200 mg bid for 20 days
Enterobius vermicularis	*Mebendazole* 100 mg once, repeated after 3 and 6 weeks. In re-infection, treat the whole family or cluster at the same time. Hygienic measures	*Pyrvinium* 5 mg base/kg once, or *Pyrantel* 10 mg base/kg once as suspension or tablet. repeated after 3 and 6 weeks
Hookworms	*Mebendazole* 100 mg tid for 3 days	1. *Albendazole* 200 mg/d for 3 days 2. *Pyrantel Embonate* 10 mg/kg/d for 3 days
Oesophagostoma bifurcum	*Albendazole* 5 mg/kg bid for 5 days	
Strongyloides stercoralis	*Ivermectin* 0.2 mg/kg/d for 2 days Hyperinfection syndrome: *Ivermectine* 0.2–0.4 mg/kg/d for 2 days, repeated after 2 weeks. Sometimes higher doses, longer therapy duration and/or combination with *Albendazole* required	1. *Albendazole* 400 mg bid, for 3 days 2. *Mebendazole* 200 mg tid for 3 days

Toxocara catis/canis **Cutaneous larva migrans**	Topical application of *Albendazole* 2% (1g) + Triamcinolone-acetonide 0,1% (0.05g) + Unguentum emulsificans aquosum ad 50.0 bid for 7–10 days	*Albendazole* 400 mg/d, for 1–3 days
Visceral larva migrans	*Albendazole* 7.5 mg/kg/d bid for 5 days CAVE: do not treat before exclusion of ocular toxocariasis. In case of ocular toxocariasis this must be treated by an experienced ophthalmologist! Cortico-steroids may be required to mitigate allergical phenomena during antiparasitic therapy	1. *Ivermectin* 0.2 mg/kg once or 2. *Diethylcarbamazine* 0.5mg/kg/d increasing to-3mg/kg/d during 7 days
Trichinella spiralis	*Prednisone* 40–60 mg/kg/d for 3–5 days than tapered + *Albendazole* 7.5 mg/kg bid for 6 days	*Prednisone* 40–60 mg/kg/d for 3–5 days than tapered + *Mebendazole* 200–400 mg tid for 3 days, than 400–500 mg/d for 10 days
***Trichostrongylus* spp.**	*Mebendazole* 100 mg tid for 3 days	1. *Levamisole* 2.5 mg/kg once or 2. *Pyrantel Embonate* 10 mg/kg/d for 3 days
Trichuris trichiura.	*Mebendazole* 100 mg bid for 3–6 days	1. *Albendazole* 400 mg/d, for 3 days 2. *Oxantel* 10 mg/kg, once
***Fasciola* spp.**	*Triclabendazole* 10 mg/kg once or repeated after 12 hrs. In acute fascioliasis corticosteroids, in chronic-latent fascioliasis spasmolytics may be required	*Bithionol* 30–50 mg every other day for 10–15 doses (less effective than triclabendazole)

(continued)

Table 15.2 (Continued)

Organism	Drug of choice and dose	Alternative
Fasciolopsis buskii	*Praziquantel* 15 mg/kg once	—
Opistorchis spp.	*Praziquantel* 25 mg/kg bid for 1 day	*Praziquantel* 50 mg/kg once
Paragonimus spp.	*Triclabendazole* 10 mg/kg	*Praziquantel* 25 mg/kg tid for 3 days
Cysticercosis	*Albendazole* 7.5 mg/kg bid for 14 days. In cerebral cysticercosis coverage with corticosteroids required, anti-epileptic drugs may be necessary. In ocular cysticercosis treatment by an experienced oculist. Antiparasitic treatment may worsen ocular cysticercosis	*Praziquantel* 50 mg/kg/d in 3 divided doses for 15 days
Giardiasis (see table1)	*Mebendazole* 200 mg tid, for 3–5 days	*Albendazole* 10–15 mg/kg/d for 3 days

tract (Richter *et al.*, 1999). Since triclabendazole is administered only as a one-day therapy in humans, data on long-term toxicity are available only from animal studies: in long-term administration to rodents during the entire life-span, the most important side effect of triclabendazole administration were benign adenomata after two years (WHO, 1993). All benzimidazoles are pregnancy category C. In animals such as rats and rabbits mebendazole and albendazole have been found to be embryotoxic and teratogenic at high doses. Although widely used even during unexpected pregnancy, embryotoxic or teratogenic effects have never been observed in humans. The level of excretion into breast milk is unknown.

Imidazole derivatives with generic and brand names

Mebendazole: Vermox, Surfont
Albendazole: Zentel, Eskazole
Triclabendazole: Egaten, Fasinex

Ivermectin

Introduction

Avermectins are derivatives of fermentation products of the actinomycete *Streptomyces avermitilis*. Ivermectin was introduced as an antiparasitic drug in 1981, and abamectin as an agricultural pesticide and antiparasitic drug in veterinary medicine in 1985.

Mechanism of action

The mechanism of action of ivermectin is not clear. It is presumed that it acts as GABA antagonist. In filariasis ivermectin is active against microfilariae but does not affect macrofilaria. For this indication, the slow and long-lasting effect is particularly suitable in control efforts.

Clinical effectiveness

Ivermectin is active against larval stages of nematodes including microfilariae of *Wuchereria bancrofti, Brugia malayensis, Onchocera volvulus, Mansonella perstans*, as well as other nematodes such as *Strongyloides spp.*, hookworms including larval *Toxocara spp., Gnathostoma spinigerum*. Furthermore, ivermectin has proven very effective against ectoparasite infections including head- and body lice, scabies, and tungiasis (Table 15.2) (Heukelbach *et al.*, 2004)

Pharmacology

Ivermectin is the only avermectin derivative used in humans.

Toxicity

Ivermectin is very well tolerated even when several-fold doses and prolonged used are required (e.g., in *Strongyloides* hyperinfection syndrome) (Richter *et al.*, 2005). Side effects are due to allergic reactions to the antigen presentation following worm damage which in filariasis is known as "Mazzotti reaction." The Mazzotti reaction in onchocerciasis may be severe and even life-threatening when microfiaraemia is high and microfilaria are present in cerebrospinal fluid. In infections other than filariasis severe reactions have not been reported. Experience with children under 15 kg is limited. In animals without a blood-brain barrier (e.g., collie-dogs), severe CNS-toxicity has been reported. In animals, teratogenicity has not been reported in rats, but high doses were neurotoxic to the newborns during lactation. Millions of people and thousands of pregnant women have been treated in tropical countries without evidence of teratogenicity in man. Ivermectin is excreted into breast milk and may attain 30% of the plasma level, but less than 10% is estimated to be taken up by the infant and is therefore estimated as clinically insignificant (Abdi *et al.*, 1995).

Brand names

Ivermectin: Stromectol, Mectizan

Praziquantel

Introduction

Praziquantel is an antihelminthic drug initially developed for the treatment of schistosomiasis. Later it has been found to have a wide spectrum of activity against other trematodes and cestodes.

Mechanism of action

The mechansism of action of praziquantel is still not clearly understood: helminths in contact with praziquantel undergo tetanic musculature contraction but tegument vacuolization appears to be the main antihelminthic effect of praziquantel.

Pharmacology

Praziquantel is given orally. Up to 80% is absorbed, and its bioavailability is increased by food. Peak plasma levels are attained 1–3 hours after ingestion. It also crosses the blood–brain barrier, with CSF concentrations approximately 25% of that in plasma.

Clinical effectiveness

Praziquantel is highly effective against a large spectrum of flatworms (platyhelminthes) including *Taenia spp.* and trematodes such as *Schistosoma spp.* and foodborne flukes among these *Clonorchis sinensis, Opistorchis spp., Paragonimus spp., Fasciolopsis buskii* (Table 15.3).

Table 15.3 Treatment indications of praziquantel

Organism	Drug of choice and dose	Alternative
Clonorchis sinensis	*Praziquantel* 25 mg/kg bid for 1 day	*Praziquantel* 50 mg/kg once
Diphyllobotrium latum	*Praziquantel* 10 mg/kg once	*Niclosamide* 2 g once
Fasciolopsis buskii	*Praziquantel* 15 mg/kg once	—
Heterophyes spp.	*Praziquantel* 20 mg/kg once	—
Hymenolepis spp.	*Praziquantel* 25 mg/kg once	*Niclosamide* 2 g on day 1, than 1g/d on days 2–7
Opistorchis spp.	*Praziquantel* 25 mg/kg bid for 1 day	*Praziquantel* 50 mg/kg once
Paragonimus spp.	*Triclabendazole* 10 mg/kg	*Praziquantel* 25 mg/kg tid for 3 days
Schistosoma haematobium, Schistosoma intercalatum	*Praziquantel* 40 mg/kg once	*S.haematobium: Metrifonate* 7.5 mg/kg once repeated after 2 and 4 weeks
Schistosoma mansoni	*Praziquantel* 40 mg/kg once	*Oxamniquine* 15–20 mg/kg once or for 2 days
Schistosoma japonicum, Schistosoma mekongi	*Praziquantel* 30 mg/kg bid for 1 or 2 days	—
Acute schistosomiasis	*Severe cases: Prednisone* 1 mg/kg/d for 1 week, followed by 0.5 mg/kg/d, and 0.25 mg/kg/d for 1 week. In mild cases, antihistaminics may be sufficient. One day after initiation of prednisone therapy: *Praziquantel* 30 mg/kg bid for 1 or 2 days, repeated after 6 weeks	*Artesunate* 50 mg bid, for 5 days (usually not sufficient if therapy is not combined with praziquantel)
Taenia spp.	*Praziquantel* 10 mg/kg once	*Niclosamide* 2 g once
Cysticercosis	*Albendazole* 7.5 mg/kg bid for 14 days. In cerebral cysticercosis coverage with corticosteroids required, anti-epileptic drugs may be necessary. In ocular cysticercosis treatment by an experienced oculist. Antiparasitic treatment may worsen ocular cysticercosis	*Praziquantel* 50 mg/kg/d in 3 divided doses for 15 days

Toxicity

Praziquantel is usually well tolerated. The most important side effects are due to immune reaction to antigen presentation following the worm damage. This is especially important to bear in mind in patients with acute or early schistosomiasis. Therefore, if possible praziquantel therapy should either been postponed, until schistosomes are mature and more susceptible to the drug, or accompanied by corticosteroids. In an expert meeting organized by WHO, fetal toxicity was considered lower than the harm directly or indirectly caused to the fetus by schistosomiasis (WHO 2002).

Brand names

Praziquantel: Biltricide, Cesol, Cysticide

Treatment dosages (Table 15.3)

Pyrvinium embonate (*syn.* pyrvinium pamoate)

Pyrvinium embonate is a quarternary ammonium derivative which may given as a suspension and is therefore an alternative for treating enterobiasis in small children from the age of 4 months on. It is effective at a single dose of 5 mg base/kg. As in all treatments of enterobiasis strict hygienic measures and simultaneous treatment of all family/cluster members are required to prevent reinfection. In case of reinfection, repetition of treatment after 3 and 6 months is recommended. Pyrvinium appears not to be absorbed systemically in humans, and is probably safe in pregnancy, although as a general precaution it is recommended to postpone therapy until after the first trimester. Side effects include nausea, vomiting, abdominal discomfort and rarely allergy or photosensitivity. Patients should be warned that stool is stained bright red by the compound and may stain clothing.

Pyrantel and oxantel

Pyrantel as well as oxantel are pyrimidine derivatives widely used in veterinary medicine. Pyrantel may be used for enterobiasis from the age of 7 months on. Oxantel is not yet approved for human use. For indications and dosages see table. Having been widely used for decades and being poorly absorbed systemically, pyrantel is probably safe in pregnancy. As a general precaution, however, it is recommended to postpone therapy until after the first trimester (Table 15.4).

Other antihelminthic drugs

Indications of other drugs with antiparasitic activity are listed in Table 15.5.

Table 15.4 Second line antihelminthic drugs

Drug	Organism	Recommended dose
Pyrvinium	*Enterobius vermicularis*	5 mg base/kg once, or repeated after 3 and 6 weeks. In re-infection, treat the whole family or cluster at the same time. Hygienic measures
Pyrantel Embonate	*Enterobius vermicularis* *Trichostrongylus spp.*	10 mg base/kg once as suspension or tablet, repeated after 3 and 6 weeks in *E vermicularis* infection. In re-infection, treat the whole family or cluster at the same time. Hygienic measures
Pyrantel Embonate	Hookworms	10 mg/kg/d for 3 days
Diethylcarbamazine (DEC)	*Toxocara catis/ canis* Visceral larva migrans	0.5 mg/kg/d increasing to-3 mg/kg/d during 7 days. In case of ocular toxocariasis this must be treated by an experienced ophthalmologist! Cortico-steroids may be required to mitigate allergical phenomena during antiparasitic therapy
Levamisole	*Trichostrongylus spp.*	2.5 mg/kg, once
Oxantel	*Trichuris trichiura*	10 mg/kg, once
Niclosamide	*Hymenolepis spp.*	2 g on day 1, than 1g/d on days 2–7
Niclosamide	*Taenia spp., Diphyllobotrium latum*	2 g once
Bithionol	*Fasciola spp.*	30–50 mg every other day for 10–15 doses (less effective than triclabendazole)
Oxamniquine	*Schistosoma mansoni*	15–20 mg/kg once or for 2 days

Table 15.5 Alternative drugs for gastrointestinal protozoal infections

Drug	Indication, susceptible organism	Dose
Paromomycin	To eradicate intestinal carriage of *Entamoeba histolytica* (*sensu stricto*)	25–35 mg/kg/d in 3 divided doses for 5–10 days
Tetracycline	*Balantidium coli, Dientamoeba fragilis*	500 mg qid for 10 days
Cotrimoxazol	*Cyclospora cayetanensis*	TMP 160 mg + SMZ 800 mg bid for 3 days
	Isospora belli	TMP 160 mg + SMZ 800 mg qid, for 10 days followed by TMP 160 mg + SMZ 800 mg bid for 20 days
Chloroquine (salt)	*Multiresistent infection by* **Giardia intestinalis** *Invasive* **Entamoeba histolytica** Colitis, amoeboma, extraintestinal amebiasis, liver abscess	10 mg/kg bid for 5 days of 250 mg bid for 7–20 days 250 mg bid for 7–20 days
Diloxanid furoate	Intestinal carriage of *Entamoeba histolytica*	500 mg tid for 10 days
Iodoquinol	*Balantidium coli, Blastocystis hominis, Dientamoeba fragilis*	650 mg tid for 20 days
Nitazoxanide	*Cryptospora parvum* Multiresistent *Giardia intestinalis* infection	500 mg/d bid, for 3 days 500 mg/d bid, for 3 days
Fumagillin	*E. bieneusi*	20 mg tid, 2 weeks

Sources: Abdi *et al.*, 1995; Molina *et al.*, 2002; Armadi *et al*, 2002; Gilles *et al.*, 2002, Escobedo *et al.*, 2007; Peréz Molina *et al.*, 2011.

Recommended reading

Abdi YA, Gustafsson LL, Ericsson Ö, Hellgren U (1995) *Handbook for Tropical Parasitic Infections*, 2nd edn. London: Taylor & Francis.
   Excellent systematic textbook on drugs for human parasitic infections. Still applicable in many respects, since all drugs used in parasitology have been developed many years ago.
Armadi B, Mwiya M, Musuku J, Watuka A, Sianongo S, Ayoub A, Kelly P (2002) Effect of nitazoxanide on morbidity and mortality in Zambian children with cryptosporidiosis: a randomised controlled trial. *Lancet* **360**: 1375–80.

Bansal D, Malla N, Mahajan RC (2006) Drug resistance in amoebiasis. *Indian J Med Res* Feb.; **123**(2): 115–18.

Blessmann J, Tannich E (2003) Treatment of asymptomatic intestinal *Entamoeba histolytica* infection. *NEJM* 1384.

Brunetti E, Kern P, Vuitton DE (2010) Writing panel for the WHO-International Working Group on Echinococcosis. Expert consensus for the diagnosis and treatment of cystic and alveolar echinococcosis in humans. *Acta Tropica* **114**: 1–16.

Datry A, Hilmasrsdottir I, Mayorga-Sagastume R, Lyagoubi M, Gaxotte P, Biligui S, Chodakewitz J, Neu D, Danis M, Gentilini M (1994) Treatment of *Strongyloides stercoralis* infection with ivermectin compared with albendazole; results of an open study of 60 cases. *Trans R Soc Trop Med Hyg* **88**: 344–5.

De Clercq D, Vercruysse J, Verle P, Niasse F, Kongs A, Diop M (2000) Efficacy of artesunate against *Schistosoma mansoni* infections in Richard Toll, Senegal. *Trans R Soc Trop Med Hyg* **94**: 90–1.

Eckert J, Deplazes D, Kern P. (2011) Alveolar echinococcosis (*Echinococcus multilocularis*) and neotropical forms of echinococcosis (*Echinococcus vogeli* and *Echinococcus oligarthrus*). In SR Palmer Lord Soulsby, PR Torgerson, DWW Brown (eds), *Oxford Textbook of Zoonoses*. Oxford: Oxford University Press, pp. 669–99.

Escobedo AA, Cimerman S. Giardiasis (2007) A pharmacotherapy review. *Expert Opin Pharmacother* **12**: 1885–1902.
Excellent and exhaustive review on all therapy attempts in giardiasis.

Gilles HM, Hoffman PS (2002) Treatment of intestinal parasitic infections: a review of nitazoxanide. *Trends Parasitol* Mar.; **18**(3): 95–7.

Heukelbach J, Winter B, Wilcke T, *et al.* (2004) Mass treatment to control helminthiasis and skin diseases. *Bull World Health Organ* **82**: 563–71.

Keiser J, Utzinger J (2004) Chemotherapy for major food-borne trematodes: a review. *Expert Opin Pharmacother* Aug; **5**(8): 1711–26.

Keiser J, Engels D, Büscher G, Utzinger J (2005) Triclabendazole for the treatment of fascioliasis and paragonimiasis. *Expert Opinion Invest Drugs* **14**(12): 1513–26.
Excellent review of therapy of flukes with triclabendazole.

Mairiang E, Mairiang P (2003) Clinical manifestations of opistorchiasis and treatment. *Acta Trop* **88**: 221–7.

Millán JC, Mull R, Freise S, Richter J, and the Triclabendazole Study Group (2000) Efficacy and tolerability of triclabendazole for the treatment of latent and chronic fascioliasis. *Am J Trop Med Hyg* **63**: 264–9.

Molina JM, Tourneur M, Sarfati C, Chevret S, de Gouvello A, Gobert JG, Balkan S, Derouin F; Agence Nationale de Recherches sur le SIDA 090 Study Group (2002) Fumagillin treatment of intestinal microsporidiosis. *N Engl J Med* June; **346**(25): 1963–9.

Peréz-Molina JA, Diaz-Menendez M, Gallego JI, Norman F, Monge-Maillo B, Peréz-Ayala A, López-Vélez R (2011) Evaluation of nitazoxanide for the treatment of disseminated cystic echinococcosis. Report of five cases and literature review. *Am J Trop Med H* **84**(2): 351–6.

Reuter S, Buck A, Grebe O, Nüssle-Kügele K, Kern P, Manfras B (2003) Salvage treatment with amphotericin B in progressive human alveolar echinococcosis. *Antimicrob Agents Chemother* **47**(11): 3586–91.

Richter D, Richter J, Grüner B, Kranz K, Franz J, Kern P (2013) In vitro efficacy of triclabendazole and clorsulon against the larval stage of *Echinocccus multilocularis*. *Paras Res* **112**(4): 1655–60.

Richter J, Freise S, Mull R, Millán JC, and the Triclabendazole Clinical Study Group (1999) Fascioliasis: sonographic abnormalities of the biliary tract and evolution after treatment with triclabendazole. *Trop Med Intern Health* **4**(11): 774–81.

Richter J, Schwarz U, Duwe S, Ellerbrok H, Poggensee G, Pauli G (2005) Recurrent strongyloidiasis as an indicator of HTLV infection [*Rezidivierende Strongyloidose als Indikator einer HTLV-infektion*]. *Dtsch Med Wochenschr* **130**: 1007–10.

World Health Organization (1993) Evaluation of certain veterinary drug residues in food. *WHO Tech Rep Ser* **832**: 1–62.

World Health Organization (2002) Report of the WHO informal consultation on the use of praziquantel during pregnancy and lactation and of albendazole and mebendazole in children under 24 months. WHO/CDS/CPE/PVC/2002.4. www.who.int. World Health Organization Geneva, Switzerland.
Evaluation and final statement of the World Health Organization on the use of praziquantel and benzimidazoles during pregnancy and lactation

World Health Organization (2007) *WHO Informal Working Group on Echinococcosis* (2007) World Health Organization Geneva, Switzerland.

CHAPTER 16
Vaccines for viral hepatitides

Savio John[1] and Raymond T. Chung[2]
[1]SUNY Upstate, Syracuse, NY, USA
[2]Harvard Medical School, Boston, MA, USA

Hepatitis A vaccination

Introduction

Hepatitis A is a serious liver disease caused by the hepatitis A virus (HAV). It is usually spread by close personal contact or by eating or drinking contaminated food or water. Humans are the only known reservoir for HAV; hence universal vaccination could potentially lead to eradication of this disease.

Pharmacology

HAV vaccines that are currently available include formalin-inactivated vaccines with and without aluminium hydroxide an adjuvant, live attenuated vaccines, and combination vaccines for HAV with hepatitis B (Twinrix) and with typhoid (Hepatyrix). The inactivated vaccines (HAVRIX and VAQTA) and combination vaccines are the only agents currently approved for use in the United States.

Mechanism of action

Inactivated virus vaccine which offers active immunization against HAV infection.

Indications for vaccination

It is recommended that all children be vaccinated against HAV between their first and second birthdays (12 through 23 months of age) In addition, vaccine should be given to children and adolescents 2 through 18 years of age who live in states or communities where routine vaccination has been implemented because of high disease incidence. Otherwise, vaccine may be administered to children 1 year of age or older whose parents wish to protection them from HAV infection.

All unvaccinated adults at risk for infection should receive immunization as well. High-risk groups include men who have sex with

Pocket Guide to Gastrointestinal Drugs, Edited by M. Michael Wolfe and Robert C. Lowe. © 2014 John Wiley & Sons, Ltd. Published 2014 by John Wiley & Sons, Ltd.

men, injection drug users, persons with chronic liver disease, and persons who are treated with clotting factor concentrates. Additionally, those who work with HAV-infected primates or who work with HAV in research laboratories should be vaccinated, as should anyone 1 year of age and older traveling to or working in countries with high or intermediate prevalence of HAV, such as those located in Central or South America, Mexico, Asia (except Japan), Africa, and eastern Europe.

Others at higher risk of infection include members of households planning to adopt a child, or care for a newly arriving adopted child, from a country where hepatitis A is common,unvaccinated children or adolescents in communities where outbreaks of hepatitis A are occurring, and unvaccinated people who have been exposed to hepatitis A virus. The Advisory Committee on Immunization Practices (ACIP) of the Centers for Disease Control and Prevention (CDC) has also recommended HAV vaccination of adults with HIV infection and in close family contacts of index cases.

Dosing and administration
HAVRIX
Primary immunization in children and adolescents (12 months through 18 years): single dose of 720 EL.U, in 0.5 mL and a booster dose (720 EL.U in 0.5 mL) any time between 6 and 12 months later.

Adults: single dose of 1440 EL.U in 1 mL and a booster dose (1440 EL.U in 1 mL) anytime between 6 and 12 months later.

VAQTA
Primary immunization in children and adolescents (12 months through 18 years): single 0.5 mL (~25 U) dose and a booster dose of 0.5 mL (~25 U) 6 to 18 months later.

Adults 19 and older: single 1.0 mL (~50 U) dose and a booster of 1.0 mL (~50 U) 6 to 18 months later.

Note
When used for primary immunization, the vaccine should be given 1 month (at least 2 weeks) prior to expected HAV exposure. Some protection may still result if the vaccine is given on or closer to the potential exposure date. When used prior to an international adoption, the vaccination series should begin when adoption is being planned, but ideally ≥2 weeks prior to expected arrival of adoptee. When used for post exposure prophylaxis, the vaccine should be given as soon as possible. Vaccines may not be effective if administered during periods of altered immune competence (CDC, 2011).

Co-administration of vaccines: The inactivated hepatitis A vaccine can be given concurrently with the other pediatric vaccines as well as with pneumococcus, typhoid, cholera, Japanese encephalitis, rabies, or yellow fever vaccines without compromising the immunogenicity or safety. The injections should be given at different sites. Preterm infants should be vaccinated at the same chronological age as full-term infants (CDC, 2011).

Administration
Vaccines should be administered intramuscularly; the deltoid is the preferred site in adults while the vastus lateralis (anterolateral thigh) is preferred in infants.

Adverse effects
Mild adverse effects include soreness at the injection site (about 1 out of 2 adults, and up to 1 out of 6 children), headache (about 1 out of 6 adults and 1 out of 25 children), loss of appetite (about 1 out of 12 children), and fatigue (about 1 out of 14 adults).

Serious allergic reaction or anaphylaxis is rare but does occur, and epinephrine should always be available for immediate use where vaccine is administered. Although serious adverse events such as Guillain-Barré syndrome, multiple sclerosis, encephalitis, elevated liver biochemical tests, jaundice and idiopathic thrombocytopenic purpura have been occasionally reported, their relationship to vaccination is unclear.

Contraindications
Vaccine should not be administered to persons with known hypersensitivity to hepatitis A vaccine or any component of the formulation. All hepatitis A vaccines contain alum, and some hepatitis A vaccines contain 2-phenoxyethanol. Anyone who is moderately or severely ill at the time the shot is scheduled should defer vaccination until recover, while those with a mild illness can usually receive the vaccine. Hepatitis A vaccine is not licensed for children younger than 1 year of age.

Clinical effectiveness
The immunogenicity of the vaccine is defined as an antibody concentration of >20 mIU/mL measured by ELISA, and is nearly 100% and long-lasting. Thus, there is no evidence that a hepatitis A booster vaccination after a full primary vaccination is needed in healthy individuals. Certain lots of VAQTA were recalled in 2001 due to low antigen count and inadequate protection. The individuals who received this vaccine may be tested for development of immunity. Due to the long incubation period for hepatitis A (15–50 days), immunization may not prevent infection in those with unrecognized hepatitis A infection. Patients with advanced

liver disease may not have a similar response rate and hence vaccination in patients with cirrhosis should be carried out at the earliest possible stage in the course of their disease.

Special considerations
Missed dose
In case of a missed dose, the second dose can be given without restarting the series.

Serologic testing before vaccination
As per CDC, testing of children is not indicated because of the low prevalence of infection in this age group. For adults, the decision is individualized and will be most cost-effective in adults who are from geographic areas that have a high or intermediate endemicity of HAV and in groups that have a high prevalence of infection (e.g., injection drug users and adults older than 40 years).

Post vaccination testing:
Post vaccination testing is not required because of the high rate of vaccine response among healthy adults and children.

Post exposure prophylaxis
As per ACIP recommendations, nonvaccinated persons who have been exposed recently to HAV should be administered a single dose of single-antigen HAV vaccine or immune globulin (IG) (0.02 mL/kg) as soon as possible. For healthy persons aged 12 months to 40 years, HAV vaccine is preferred. For children aged <12 months, immunocompromised persons, persons who have had chronic liver disease diagnosed, and persons for whom vaccine is contraindicated, IG is recommended.

Pregnancy class
Pregnancy risk factor: C.
Inactivated vaccines have not been shown to cause increased risks to the fetus (CDC, 2011 Inactivated vaccines such as HAV do not affect the safety of breast-feeding for the mother or the infant (CDC, 2011).

Hepatitis B vaccination (Table 16.1)

Introduction
The worldwide prevalence of hepatitis B virus (HBV) infection based on serologic tests is estimated to be in excess of 2 billion. The annual mortality from chronic hepatitis B related cirrhosis and hepatocellular carcinoma (HCC) is between half a million to 1.2 million. Each year about

Table 16.1 Hepatitis B vaccine types with brand names

Vaccine	Type	Manufacturing country
Recombivax HB®	Yeast-derived recombinant	USA
Engerix-B®	Yeast-derived recombinant	USA
Twinrix®	Combination of Engerix-B® and HAVRIX® (HAV vaccine)	USA
Comvax®	Haemophilus b conjugate/ HBV recombinant vaccine	USA
Pediarix®	Diphtheria/tetanus toxoids and acellular pertussis/hepatitis B/ poliovirus, inactivated vaccine	USA
Gen Hevac B	Mammalian cell-derived	France
Bio-Hep-B/Sci-B-Vac	Mammalian cell-derived	Israel
AG-3	mammalian cell-derived	UK

2000–4000 people die in the United States from cirrhosis or hepatocellular carcinoma caused by HBV. HBV is spread through contact with the blood or other body fluids of an infected person, but people can also be infected from contact with a contaminated object, where the virus can live for up to 7 days. The World Health Organization has strongly advocated hepatitis B vaccination with the goal of eradicating HBV, especially given the extreme safety, excellent efficacy and pangenotypic action profile of hepatitis B vaccine.

Pharmacology

There are three different classes of hepatitis B vaccine, i.e., vaccine derived from plasma, yeast, or mammalian cells. The first generation vaccine was prepared by concentrating and purifying plasma from Hepatitis B surface antigen (HBsAg) carriers to produce 22 nm subviral particles that contain only HBsAg. Due to the potential for transmitting blood-borne infections and the marginal difference in cost with the newer generation vaccines, these vaccines are no longer used. Yeast-derived recombinant Hepatitis B vaccines are produced by cloning of the HBV S gene in yeast cells. These vaccines do not contain antigens of the pre-S regions. The original preparations of this vaccine contained an inorganic mercurial, thimerosal, used as a preservative, which carries a potential risk for abnormal neurodevelopment in children. Hence thimerosal-free yeast-derived recombinant vaccines have been developed, of which Recombivax HB®

and Engerix-B® are available in the U.S. The newer mammalian cell-derived recombinant vaccines contain antigen from the pre-S2 region or antigens from both the pre-S1 and pre-S2 regions. Although these vaccines provide enhanced immunologic response, they are not widely available. A combination vaccine (Twinrix®), including Engerix-B and HAVRIX (hepatitis A vaccine), has been approved for use in adults in the United States and Europe, and in children in some countries. Hepatitis B vaccine is also available as multivalent vaccines in combination with diphtheria, tetanus, pertussis, and *Haemophilus influenzae* type B and is widely used in childhood immunization programs with increased compliance and reduced cost.

Mechanism of action

Recombinant hepatitis B vaccine is a noninfectious subunit viral vaccine, derived from HB$_s$Ag via recombinant DNA techniques from yeast cells. This vaccine confers active immunity via formation of antihepatitis B surface (anti-HBs) antibodies.

Indications for vaccination

It is recommended that all children and adolescents be vaccinated against HBV, and anyone up to 18 years of age who did not previously receive the vaccine should also be immunized.

Unvaccinated adults at risk for HBV infection should be vaccinated as well. This group includes the sex partners of people infected with HBV, men who have sex with men, injection drug users, and those with more than one sex partner. Vaccination is also recommended for people with chronic liver or kidney disease and those under 60 years of age with diabetes, people with jobs that expose them to human blood or other body fluids, household contacts of people infected with hepatitis B, residents and staff in institutions for the developmentally disabled, chronic hemodialysis patients, travelers to countries where HBV is endemic, and those with HIV infection.

The American Association for the Study of Liver Diseases (AASLD) recommends vaccination for the following groups as well: pregnant women, United States-born persons not vaccinated as infants whose parents were born in regions with high HBV endemicity, persons with chronically elevated aminotransferases, persons needing immunosuppressive therapy, inmates of correctional facilities, HCV-infected patients, and sexual contacts of HBV-infected persons. The Advisory Committee on Immunization Practices (ACIP) recommends vaccination for any persons who are wounded in bombings or similar mass casualty events who have penetrating injuries or nonintact skin exposure, or who have contact with mucous membranes (exception – superficial contact with intact skin), and who cannot confirm receipt of a hepatitis B vaccination (Chapman *et al.*, 2008).

Dosing and administration

Adults and children >10 years: I.M.: 1 mL/dose (adult formulation) of Engerix-B or Recombivax HB for 3 total doses administered at 0, 1, and 6 months.

    Infants and children up to 10 years: 0.5 mL/dose (pediatric/adolescent formulation) for 3 total doses administered at birth or zero months, 1 and 6 months.

Note:

The second and third doses may be given at 1–2 months of age and 6–18 months of age respectively. If a combination vaccine is used, some infants might get an extra fourth dose, which is not harmful. Neonates of HBsAg positive mothers should be given HBIG as well as HB vaccine at two different sites within 12 hours of delivery. Combination vaccines (e.g., vaccines containing Hepatitis B with DTaP, HIB) should not be used for the "birth" dose but may be used to complete the course beginning after the infant is ≥6 weeks of age. Premature neonates <2 kg may have the initial dose deferred up to 30 days of chronological age or at hospital discharge (CDC, 2005).

    Though the concentration (mcg/ml) of the two adult and pediatric vaccines are different, the effective dose is the same when dosed in terms of volume (both 1 mL). It is possible to interchange the vaccines for completion of a series or for booster doses; the antibody produced in response to each type of vaccine is comparable, however, the quantity of the vaccine will vary.

Administration

Vaccines should be administered intramuscularly; the deltoid is the preferred site in adults while the vastus lateralis (anterolateral thigh) is preferred in infants.

Adverse effects

Mild side effects include soreness at the injection site (about 1 person in 4) and a temperature of 99.9 °F or higher (about 1 person in 15). Severe allergic reactions (difficulty breathing, hoarseness or wheezing, hives, paleness, weakness, a fast heart beat, dizziness, high fever or unusual behavior) are rare and may occur about once in 1.1 million doses. Anaphylaxis is rare but does occur, and epinephrine should always be available for immediate use The vaccine contains noninfectious material, which cannot cause hepatitis B infection.

Contraindications

HBV vaccine should not be given to anyone with a life-threatening allergy to yeast, or to any other component of the vaccine or who has had a life-threatening allergic reaction to a previous dose of hepatitis B vaccine. Anyone who is moderately or severely ill should defer vaccination until recovery.

Clinical effectiveness

Vaccination provides a response rate close to 95% in healthy individuals. Although anti-HBs titers decrease with time, the duration of protection persists for up to 22 years after the primary vaccination schedule. Despite declining anti-HBs levels over time, the priming of memory cells with the initial vaccination produces an anamnestic response when challenged. In the US, a booster dose is not recommended for adults with normal immune status, although this varies in different countries. In patients on hemodialysis, it is generally agreed to monitor anti-HBs levels annually and consider booster dose if the levels are <10 mIU/mL[3]. Due to the long incubation period for hepatitis B, immunization may not prevent HBV infection in patients with unrecognized hepatitis B infection.

Special considerations

Missed dose

An interruption in the vaccination schedule does not require revaccination with the entire series of vaccination or addition of extra doses. In case of a missed second dose, it should be administered as soon as possible and if the third dose is delayed, it should be administered when convenient. The second and third doses should be separated by an interval of at least two months.

Pre-vaccination screening

In non-endemic areas, pre-vaccination screening is unnecessary in low-risk patient groups as the costs of screening will be much higher than the savings on the vaccine. In endemic areas, pre-vaccination screening not only provides a cost-effective strategy, but also helps identifying infected patients who might benefit from treatment, given the high prevalence of current or past infection of more than 50% in such areas. Although testing for anti-HBc alone will detect individuals with past or current infection in endemic areas, the potential for false positive test results and the benefits of identification of HBV carriers favor an approach of testing for HBsAg and anti-HBs in such individuals.

Vaccination strategy based on available results

Patients with serologic markers of past infection (positive anti-HBc and anti-HBs) do not need HBV vaccination as they will be able to mount an appropriate immune response to a new infection, even with low titers of anti-HBs. Individuals with isolated anti-HBc (negative HBsAg and anti-HBs) will need full vaccination, if they are from a low endemic area and have no risk factors for HBV.

Post vaccination testing

Routine post-vaccination testing to document anti-HBs seroconversion is unnecessary in healthy individuals. The response rate is considerably lower in immunosuppressed patient, organ transplant recipients, children with celiac disease and patients with cirrhosis or chronic renal failure. Post vaccination testing is suggested in health-care workers, patients on chronic hemodialysis, and other individuals who are at risk for recurrent exposure to hepatitis B. Testing should be done one to two months after completion of the primary vaccination series, except for infants born to HBsAg positive mothers in whom testing should only be performed at age 9 to 15 months. Those with anti-HBs levels less than 10 mIU/mL (nonresponders) should be given a repeat three-dose vaccination. Individuals who fail to respond after the repeat vaccination series are unlikely to benefit from further vaccination. These individuals, however, may still mount an adequate immune response and recover from HBV infection. Those with suboptimal anti-HBs level after a repeat vaccination series should be tested for HBsAg and anti-HBc.

Pregnancy class

Pregnancy Risk Factor: C.
The vaccine has no teratogenic potential and is safe in pregnancy. Pregnancy itself is not a contraindication to vaccination; vaccination should be considered if otherwise indicated (CDC, 2006). Excretion of vaccine components in breast milk is unknown. Breast-feeding infants should be vaccinated according to the recommended schedules (CDC, 2011).

Recommended reading

Advisory Committee on Immunization Practices (ACIP), Fiore AE, Wasley A, Bell BP (2006) Prevention of hepatitis A through active or passive immunization: recommendations of the Advisory Committee on Immunization Practices (ACIP). *MMWR Recomm Rep* May; **55**(RR-7): 1–23.

Centers for Disease Control and Prevention (CDC) (2005) A comprehensive immunization strategy to eliminate transmission of hepatitis B virus infection in the United States: Recommendations of the Advisory Committee on Immunization Practices (ACIP) Part I: Immunization of Infants, Children, and Adolescents, *MMWR Recomm Rep*, **54**(RR-16): 1–23.

Centers for Disease Control and Prevention (CDC) (2006) A comprehensive immunization strategy to eliminate transmission of hepatitis B virus infection in the

United States: Recommendations of the Advisory Committee on Immunization Practices (ACIP) Part II: Immunization of Adults, *MMWR Recomm Rep*, **54** (RR-16): 1–25.

Centers for Disease Control and Prevention (CDC) (2011) Recommendations of the Advisory Committee on Immunization Practices (ACIP): General Recommendations on Immunization, *MMWR Recomm Rep*, **60**(2): 1–64.

Chapman LE, Sullivent EE, Grohskopf LA, *et al.* (2008) Recommendations for postexposure interventions to prevent infection with hepatitis B virus, hepatitis C virus, or human immunodeficiency virus, and tetanus in persons wounded during bombings and other mass-casualty events – United States, 2008: Recommendations of the Centers for Disease Control and Prevention (CDC). *MMWR Recomm Rep*, **57**(RR-6): 1–21.

Edey M, Barraclough K, Johnson DW (2010) Review article: Hepatitis B and dialysis. *Nephrology (Carlton)* Mar; **15**(2): 137–45.

Lemon SM, Thomas DL (1997) Vaccines to prevent viral hepatitis. *N Engl J Med* Jan.; **336**(3): 196–204.

Lok AS, McMahon BJ (2009) Chronic hepatitis B: update 2009. *Hepatology* Sep.; **50**(3): 661–2.

Vaccine Information Statement (Interim). Hepatitis A Vaccine 10/25/2011.

Vaccine Information Statement (Interim). Hepatitis B Vaccine. 2/2/2012.

Van Damme P, Banatvala J, Fay O, Iwarson S, McMahon B, Van Herck K, Shouval D, Bonanni P, Connor B, Cooksley G, Leroux-Roels G, Von Sonnenburg F; International Consensus Group on Hepatitis A Virus Immunity (2003) Hepatitis A booster vaccination: is there a need? *Lancet* Sep.; **362**(9389): 1065–71.
This paper reports the consensus opinion that HAV booster is not needed after primary immunization.

CHAPTER 17
Rotavirus and other enteric vaccinations

Christopher J. Moran and Esther J. Israel

Mass General Hospital for Children, Boston, MA, USA

Rotavirus vaccination

Introduction

Rotavirus is a double-stranded RNA virus that is serotyped by its gly-coprotein (G) and protease-sensitive protein (P) types. The majority of rotaviral infections in the United States are due to the P[8]G1 strain (78%) and the P[4]G2 strain accounts for 9%, with the remaining 13% consisting of numerous other strains.

Infection with rotavirus causes gastroenteritis leading to severe dehydration. Symptoms in the initial 24 hours include high fever and vomiting, and usually culminate in severe diarrhea. Severe episodes of gastroenteritis are most prevalent in young children, with nearly 1 in every 50 children worldwide being hospitalized for rotavirus by 5 years of age. The principal season of rotaviral infections begins in the south-western United States in December and reaches its peak in northeastern United States in late April to May.

Pharmacology

There are two currently available rotaviral vaccines. One is a monovalent vaccine (RV1 – Rotarix) that contains a single rotavirus strain (G1P1A[8]). The other, a pentavalent vaccine (RV5 – Rotateq) includes four rotavi-ruses composed of human outer capsid proteins (G1, G2, G3, G4) and the bovine P7[5] attachment protein and one additional rotavirus with the human P1A[8] attachment protein and a bovine outer capsid protein. Both RV1 and RV5 are approved for use in the United States.

Mechanism of action

RV1 and RV5 are orally-administered, inactivated-viral vaccines that result in active immunization against rotavirus.

Pocket Guide to Gastrointestinal Drugs, Edited by M. Michael Wolfe and Robert C. Lowe. © 2014
John Wiley & Sons, Ltd. Published 2014 by John Wiley & Sons, Ltd.

Indications for vaccination

Children are particularly vulnerable to rotavirus infection and experience the greatest morbidity. Thus, the vaccine is suggested for all infants with the first dose given between 2 months to 14 weeks and 6 days.

Dosing and administration

RV5 (Rotateq)

Primary immunization: single 2 mL dose is supplied in single-dose squeezable tube/applicator. The standard schedule for RV5 is at ages 2, 4, and 6 months (with ≥4 weeks between doses). The series must be completed by 8 months of life as it has not been studied in older infants.

RV1 (Rotarix)

Primary immunization: single 1 mL dose is reconstituted from lyophilized vaccine and diluent. The standard schedule for RV1 is at ages 2 and 4 months (with ≥4 weeks between doses). The series must be completed by 8 months of life as it has not been studied in older infants.

Co-administration of vaccines: Rotaviral vaccine can be given concurrently with the other pediatric vaccines.

Preterm infants can be vaccinated as early as 6 weeks of age if healthy (such as at the time of hospital discharge). They should be vaccinated at the same chronological age as full-term infants.

Note: The rotaviral vaccine series should be completed using the same product, although unavailability of the desired product should not prevent completion of the series with the alternate product.

Adverse effects

A rhesus-based tetravalent vaccine (RRV-TV, Rotashield) was licensed for use in 1998 to prevent severe rotaviral gastroenteritis. Post-licensing analysis revealed a 20-fold increased risk of intussusception in the 2 weeks after immunization with the estimated risk to be close to 1 case of intussusception per 10 000 vaccinated infants. As a result, RRV-TV was taken off the market.

Large-scale trials in the United States did not show an increased risk of intussusception for the currently available rotavirus vaccines. However, analysis of national health registries in Australia, Brazil, and Mexico suggest that both RV1 and RV5 vaccines may confer a small increased risk of intussusception although significantly less than the data from RRV-TV. Preliminary analysis of post-marketing reports in the United States have not shown any increased risk for either RV1 or RV5. RV5 vaccination resulted in increased rates (compared to placebo) of the following adverse effects: diarrhea (24.1% vs. 21.3%), vomiting (15.2% vs. 13.6%), otitis media (14.5% vs. 13.0%) nasopharyngitis (6.9% vs. 5.8%), and bronchospasm (1.1% vs. 0.7%).

Serious allergic reactions have rarely been reported. Kawasaki's disease has been reported following both RV1 and RV5 administration but the possibility of increased risk have not reached statistical significance in large studies.

Contraindications

Vaccine should not be administered to persons with known hypersensitivity to any vaccine component or previous anaphylaxis to the vaccine. It should be noted that the RV1 applicator contains latex and should not be used to vaccinate infants with latex allergy; the RV5 vaccine system does not contain latex. While infants living with pregnant women and immunocompromised people may receive the Rotavirus vaccine, precautions (with comparison of risks and benefits) should be taken in infants with an immunocompromising illness moderate to severe acute illness (those with mild illness may receive rotavirus vaccine), chronic gastrointestinal disease. bladder exstrophy and spina bifida (due to high risk of latex allergy), or a history of intussusception.

Clinical effectiveness

Rotavirus vaccine has clearly decreased the incidence of gastroenteritis in infants. RV1 vaccine reduced the incidence of severe rotaviral gastroenteritis from 13.3 to 2.0 per 1000 infant-years). The greatest protection was seen in the G1P[8] serotype (that was the basis for the vaccine), although protection was also demonstrated for G3P[8], G4P[8], G9P[8], and G2P[4] serotypes.

RV5 vaccine has been shown to reduce rotaviral gastroenteritis-associated hospitalizations by 95.8% and rotaviral gastroenteritis-associated ER visits by 93.7%. Cases of G1-G4 rotavirus gastroenteritis were reduced by 74.0% while severe G1–G4 cases were reduced by 98%. In subgroup analysis, 95.2% of immunized patients had antirotavirus IgA seroconversion compared to 14.3% of placebo.

Special considerations

Vaccination in those receiving blood products

Infants who have received recent blood transfusions or antibody-containing products may be vaccinated per standard recommendations.

Post-exposure vaccination

If an infant is exposed to rotavirus before completion of the full vaccination series, the series should be resumed per standard recommendations (but subjects with moderate to severe acute gastroenteritis should wait until the episode has resolved).

Typhoid fever vaccination

Introduction

Typhoid fever is an enteric infection caused by the Gram-negative bacterium, *Salmonella typhi*. Typhoid fever, combined with the similar condition paratyphoid fever (caused by S. paratyphoid A and B), comprise the syndrome of enteric fever. Symptoms of enteric fever are recurrent fevers, abdominal pain, and headaches. The most recent global analysis cited 27 million cases of typhoid fever per year with 200 000 deaths (mostly occurring in children). Despite these high numbers, only 400 cases are reported in the United States per year with the majority occurring in US citizens traveling to endemic areas.

Pharmacology

There are two currently available typhoid fever vaccines. One is an attenuated Salmonella bacterium (Ty21a – Vivotif). The other is a purified Salmonella capsular antigen (ViCPS, Typherix, Typhi Vi).

Mechanism of action

Ty21a is an orally-administered, highly-attenuated Vi-negative *S. typhi* strain that results in active immunization against *S. typhi*. Vaccination also results in some cross-protection against *S. paratyphi* B (but not *S. paratyphi* A).

ViCPS is an injectable Vi capsular polysaccharide antigen from *S. typhi* that results in active immunization against *S. typhi*. ViCPS does not offer cross-protection against *S. paratyphi*.

Indications for vaccination

Individuals travelling to endemic areas should be vaccinated. Typhoid fever vaccines are not a part of routine childhood vaccine schedules, but travelers ≥2 years old may receive ViCPS and those ≥5 years old may receive Ty21a.

Dosing and administration

Ty21a

Primary immunization: Oral dose given every 2 days for 4 total doses. The vaccine course should be completed 1 week prior to travel.

ViCPS

Primary immunization: Single intramuscular injection that should be given 2 weeks prior to travel.

Adverse effects

The adverse effects of ViCPS immunization include fever (1%) headache (3%), and injection site reaction (6%).

Ty21a vaccine has been associated with fever or headache (5%), and abdominal pain (<1%).

Contraindications

ViCPS should not be given to children <2 years of age or to anyone who has had hypersensitivity to any vaccine component or previous anaphylaxis to the vaccine. In addition, those who are moderately or severely ill should delay vaccination until after recovery.

Ty21a is contraindicated in children <6 years of age or those with prior hypersensitivity to any vaccine component or previous anaphylaxis to the vaccine. Those whoare moderately or severely ill should delay vaccination until recovery, and those with a weakened immune system (HIV, immunosuppressant medications, cancer) should receive the ViCPS vaccine rather than Ty21a.

Clinical effectiveness

ViCPS is 70% effective at inducing protective immunity that lasts up to 3 years, while Ty21a has been shown to be 60–70% effective at inducing protective immunity that lasts up to 7 years.

Recommended reading

Centers for Disease Control and Prevention (2010) Statement Regarding Rotarix and Rotateq Rotavirus Vaccines and Intussusception. CDC. http://www.cdc.gov/vaccines/vpd-vac/rotavirus/intussusception-studies-acip.htm, Nov. 3, 2010.

Cortese MM, Parashar UD (2009) Prevention of Rotavirus Gastroenteritis among Infants and Children. Recommendations of the Advisory Committee on Immunization Practices (ACIP). *MMWR Recomm Rep* Feb.; **58**(RR02): 1–25.

Greenberg HB, Estes MK (2009) Rotaviruses: from pathogenesis to vaccination. *Gastroenterology* **136**: 1939–51.

Martin LB (2012) Vaccines for typhoid fever and other salmonellosis. *Current Opinion in Infectious Disease* Oct.; **25**(5): 489–99.
Up-to-date review of the vaccine options for the prevention of salmonellosis.

Ruiz-Palacios GM, Perez-Schael I, Velazquez FR, *et al.* (2006) Safety and efficacy of an attenuated vaccine against severe rotavirus gastroenteritis. *N Eng J Med* **354**(1): 11–22.
This double-blind, placebo-controlled trial showed that the attenuated G1P[8] human rotavirus vaccine was effective at reducing hospitalization rates and occurrence of severe rotaviral gastroenteritis. There was not an increased risk for intussusception

Vesikari T, Matson DO, Dennehy P, *et al.* (2006) Safety and efficacy of a pentavalent human-bovine (WC3) reassortant rotavirus vaccine. *N Eng J Med* **354**(1): 23–33.
This study demonstrated a >90% reduction in hospitalizations and ER visits for rotavirus in vaccinated children. This double-blind, placebo-controlled trial showed that the live pentavalent human-bovine reassortant rotavirus vaccine was effective at reducing hospitalization rates and ER visits and did not increase risk for intussusception.

NUTRITION AND PROBIOTICS

PART V

CHAPTER 18

Parenteral and enteral nutrition feeding formulas

Dominic N. Reeds[1] and Beth Taylor[2]

[1]Washington University School of Medicine, St. Louis, MO, USA
[2]Barnes-Jewish Hospital, St. Louis, MO, USA

Introduction

This chapter will provide guidelines for the general use of enteral nutrition (EN) and total parenteral nutrition as a form of nutrition support (NS) in hospitalized patients. Readers are directed to the American Society for Parenteral and Enteral Nutrition (ASPEN) guidelines for more discussion of management of critically ill, severely malnourished or pediatric patients.

Indications for nutrition support

Nutrition support is indicated when patients are unable to ingest sufficient calories and nutrients for a prolonged period of time to prevent the adverse consequences of malnutrition. Unfortunately the precise definitions of "sufficient" and "prolonged" are unclear. Several studies suggest that in most noncritically ill patients, *without* pre-existing malnutrition, NS does not improve outcomes unless the patient has failed to meet their macronutrient needs for 7–10 days. Prior to beginning any form of NS it is necessary to calculate energy requirements and macronutrient needs. In severely malnourished patients (e.g., low body mass index, >10% weight loss) early consultation with a nutrition support service is recommended.

Energy and macronutrient requirements

Energy requirements: Many formulas exist for calculating energy expenditure. A simple estimate of total daily energy requirements in hospitalized patients can be calculated based on body mass index (BMI) (Table 18.1). Hypocaloric feeding may benefit obese patients during critical illness.

Pocket Guide to Gastrointestinal Drugs, Edited by M. Michael Wolfe and Robert C. Lowe. © 2014 John Wiley & Sons, Ltd. Published 2014 by John Wiley & Sons, Ltd.

Table 18.1 Estimated energy requirements for hospitalized patients based on body mass index

BMI (kg/m^2)	Energy requirements (kcal/kg/day)
< 15	35–40
15–19	30–35
20–29	20–25
>30	15–20*

These values are recommended for critically-ill patients and all obese patients; add 20% of total calories in estimating energy requirements in noncritically-ill patients.
*The lower range within each BMI category should be considered in insulin-resistant or critically ill patients to decrease the risk of hyperglycemia and infection associated with overfeeding.
Source: Adapted from Klein (2002). Reproduced with permission of Elsevier.

Protein

Human proteins are composed of amino acids, which may be divided into essential, non-essential or conditionally-essential amino acids. 15–20% of total protein requirements should be in the form of essential amino acids. Individual protein requirements are affected by several factors, such as the amount of nonprotein calories provided, exogenous losses (e.g., chylothorax, surgical drains) and nutritional status. In patients with output from drains, the protein content of the fluid should be measured. Protein needs are affected by caloric supply, and during hypocaloric feeding, generous amounts of protein ($\geq$2.0–2.5g/kg ideal body weight/day) are needed. Protein requirements for several clinical conditions are summarized in Table 18.2.

Table 18.2 Recommended daily protein intake

Clinical condition	Protein requirements (grams / kg IBW/day)
Normal	0.75
Metabolic "stress"	1.0–1.5
Hemodialysis	1.2–1.4
Peritoneal dialysis	1.3–1.5
Continuous dialysis	1.7–2.0

IBW=ideal body weight. Males: 50 kg + 2.3 kg for each inch over 5 feet. Females: 45.5 kg + 2.3 kg for each inch over 5 feet.

Additional protein requirements are needed to compensate for excess protein loss in specific patient populations, such as patients with burn injuries, external drains and protein-losing enteropathy or nephropathy. Lower protein intake may be necessary in patients with chronic renal insufficiency not treated by dialysis.

Source: Adapted from Klein (2002). Reproduced with permission of Elsevier.

Carbohydrate

There is no dietary requirement for carbohydrate because glucose can be synthesized from precursors including amino acids. Patients with liver or renal failure may require intravenous carbohydrate during prolonged fasting or metabolic stress to prevent hypoglycemia.

Lipids

Dietary lipids are composed mainly of triglycerides: long-chain triglycerides (LCTs), which contain fatty acids that are > 12 carbons in length, or medium-chain triglycerides (MCTs), which are 6 to 12 carbons in length.

Linoleic acid (C18:2, n-6) should constitute at least 2% and linolenic acid (C18:3, n-6,9, 12) at least 0.5% of the daily caloric intake to prevent essential fatty-acid deficiency (EFAD). The plasma pattern of increased triene-tetraene ratio (>0.4) can be used to detect EFAD.

Enteral liquid feeding formulations

Formulas can be divided into four general categories: elemental formulas, semi-elemental formulas, intact-protein (polymeric) formulas, and disease-specific formulas (Table 18.3). Formula choice should be based on nutrient requirements and tolerance.

Elemental formulas consist of free amino acids, are extremely unpalatable and require tube feeding. The theoretical benefit of these formulas is that they do not require intraluminal digestion and might benefit people with exocrine pancreatic dysfunction. Absorption of elemental formulas has not been shown to be clinically superior to polymeric formulas.

Semi-elemental formulas consists of hydrolyzed protein resulting in small peptides of varying lengths (typically <40 amino acids). The potential advantage of semi-elemental formulas is related to the uptake and absorption of intact di- and tripeptides, which are absorbed more efficiently than are free amino acids or whole protein. Therefore these formulas have theoretical, but unproven, benefit in patients with limited absorptive capacity (e.g., short gut).

Intact-protein formulas consist of whole proteins, carbohydrate as glucose polymers, and lipid as LCTs or a mixture of LCTs and MCTs. These formulas can be used as a dietary supplement or can provide complete calorie, macro- and micronutrient requirements. These formulas are classified as milk-based or lactose-free.

Milk-based formulas are palatable and contain milk as a source of protein and fat. Although milk-based formulas are not recommended for lactose-intolerant patients, they can be well tolerated when given as a slow, continuous infusion.

Table 18.3 Standard enteral feeding formulas

Product	Manufacturer	Type of formula*	Oral (O) Tube (T)	Caloric distribution (%)			Caloric density (kcal/mL)	Osmolality (mOsmol/kg)	Fiber (g/1000 kcal)	Protein (g/1000 kcal)	CHO (g/1000 kcal)	Fat (g/1000 kcal)
				Protein	CHO	Fat						
Boost	Nestle	S	O	17	67	16	1	610–670	0	43	170	18
Boost HP	Nestle	HP	O	24	55	21	1	650–690	0	60.4	140	22.8
Boost Plus	Nestle	S	O	16	50	34	1.5	630–670	0	40.1	125	137.5
Boost Glucose Control	Nestle	D	O	33	34	33	0.8	400	12.4	82.5	82.5	27.8
CIB	Nestle	S	O	23	74	3	0.8	NA	0	62.5	182	2.2
CIB No Sugar added	Nestle	D	O	33	63	4	0.56	NA	0	82.5	157.5	4.4
CIB lactose free	Nestle	S	O	14	51	35	1	480	0	8.7	127	40
CIB lactose free plus	Nestle	S	O	14	47	39	1.5	620	0	35	117	43
CIB lactose free VHC	Nestle	S	O	16	34	50	2.25	950	0	40	87.8	54.6
Crucial	Nestle	IM	T	25	36	39	1.5	490	0	62.5	90	45
Diabeti-Source AC	Nestle	D	T	20	36	44	1.2	450	10	50	90	49
Ensure	Abbott	S	O,T	14.4	64	21.6	1.06	620	0	36	160	24
Ensure Plus	Abbott	S	O,T	14.8	57	28.2	1.5	680	0	37	142.5	31.3
Ensure Bone Health	Abbott	S	O	18.3	56.9	24.8	0.95	540		45.7	142	27.5
Ensure clinical strength	Abbott	S	O	15	57	28	1.5	850	0	52	142	31
Ensure Enlive	Abbott	S	O	14	86	0	1.01	796	0	28	215	0
Ensure High Protein	Abbott	HP	O,T	21	55	24	0.97	610	0	48	137.5	26.6

Ensure Immune Health	Abbott	IM	O	14	65	21	1.06	620	0	36	160	24
Ensure Muscle Health	Abbott	HP	O	21	51	28	1.06	740	0	52	127	31
Fibersource HN	Nestle	F	T	18	53	29	1.2	490	8.33	45	132.5	32
Glucerna	Abbott	D	O,T	16.7	34.3	49	1	355	14.4	41.8	93.7	55.7
Glucerna 1.2	Abbott	D	O,T	20	35	45	1.2	720	14.6	50	87.5	50
Glucerna 1.5	Abbott	D	O,T	22	33	45	1.5	876	15.2	56	82.5	50
Glucerna Shake	Abbott	D	O	20	48	32	0.84	N/A	12	50	120	35.5
Hi-Cal	Abbott	S	O	16.7	43.2	40.1	2	705	0	42	108	44
Impact	Nestle	IM	T	22	53	25	1	375	0	56	132	28
Impact with fiber	Nestle	IM	T	22	53	25	1	375	10	56	140	28
Impact 1.5	Nestle	IM	T	22	38	40	1.5	550	0	55	95	44
Impact AR	Nestle	IM	O	22	53	25	1.4	930	9.57	55	132.5	28
Impact Glutamine	Nestle	IM	T	24	46	30	1.3	630	1.9	60	115	34
Impact Peptide 1.5	Nestle	IM	T	25	37	38	1.5	510	0	62.5	92.5	43.3
Isosource 1.5	Nestle	HP	O,T	18	44	38	2	650	8	45.3	113.3	43.3
Isosource HN	Nestle	HP	T	18	52	30	1.2	490	0	44	130	34
Jevity 1 cal	Abbott	F	O,T	16.7	54.3	29	1.06	300	14.4	42	144	32.2
Jevity 1.2	Abbott	F	O,T	18.5	52.5	29	1.2	450	18	55.5	169	32.2
Jevity 1.5	Abbott	F	O,T	17	53.6	29.4	1.5	525	22	42.5	144	33
Nepro w/ carb steady	Abbott	R	O,T	18	34	48	1.8	600	8.6	45	85	53
Novasource Renal	Nestle	R	O,T	18	37	45	2	800	0	45	92.5	50
Nutren 1.0	Nestle	S	T	16	51	33	1	412	0	40	127	38

(continued)

Table 18.3 (Continued)

Product	Manufacturer	Type of formula*	Oral (O) Tube (T)	Caloric distribution (%)			Caloric density (kcal/ mL)	Osmolality (mOsmol/kg)	Fiber (g/1000 kcal)	Protein (g/1000 kcal)	CHO (g/1000 kcal)	Fat (g/1000 kcal)
				Protein	CHO	Fat						
Nutren 1.0 with Fiber	Nestle	S	O,T	16	51	33	1	310–370	14	40	127	38
Nutren 1.5	Nestle	S	O,T	16	45	39	1.5	430–530	0	40	113	45
Nutren 2.0	Nestle	S	T	16	39	45	2	745	0	40	97.5	50
Nutren Glytrol	Nestle	D	T	18	40	42	1	280	15.2	45	100	15.2
NutriHep	Nestle	L	T	11	77	12	1.5	620–650	0	26	193	14
Nutren Pulmonary	Nestle	P	O	18	27	55	1.5	450	0	45	67	63
Nutren Replete	Nestle	HP	T	25	45	30	1	290	0	37	130	35
Optimental	Abbott	PB, IM	T	20.5	55	24.5	1	540	0	51.3	138.5	28.4
Optisource HP Drink	Nestle	HP	O	49	24	27	0.85	150		122	60	30
Osmolite 1 cal	Abbott	S	T	16.7	54.3	29	1.06	300	0	42	133.6	32.2
Osmolite 1.2	Abbott	S	T	18.5	52.5	29	1.2	360	0	55.5	169	32.2
Osmolite 1.5	Abbott	S	T	16.7	54.2	29	1.5	525	0	42	135	32
Oxepa	Abbott	IM	T	16.7	28.1	55.2	1.5	535	0	45	100	47.5
Peptamen	Nestle	PB	O,T	16	51	33	1	270–380	0	40	127	39
Peptamen w / Prebio	Nestle	PB, IM	O,T	16	51	33	1	300	4	40	127	39
Peptamen AF	Nestle	PB, IM	T	25	36	39	1.2	390	0	62.5	90	43

Peptamen Bariatric	Nestle	PB, IM	T	37	30	33	1	345	0	92.5	75	37
Perative	Abbott	IM	T	20.5	55	25	1.3	460	0	51	136	29
Pivot 1.5	Abbott	PB, IM	T	25	45	30	1.5	595	5	62.5	112	33
Promote	Abbott	HP	O,T	25	52	23	1	340	0	62.5	130	26
Promote with fiber	Abbott	HP	O,T	25	50	25	1	380	14.4	62.5	139	28
Pulmocare	Abbott	P	O,T	16.7	28.1	55.2	1.5	465	0	41.7	70.4	61.4
Renalcal	Nestle	R	T	7	58	35	2	600	0	17	145	41
Resource 2.0	Nestle	HP	O	17	43	40	2	790	0	42.5	107.5	45
Resource Arginaide	Nestle	IM	O	17	83	0	1.06	1340	0	42.5	207	0
Resource Breeze	Nestle	S	O	14	86	0	1.06	750	0	35	215	0
Suplena	Abbott	R	O,T	10	42	48	1.8	600	0	25	105	53
TwoCal HN	Abbott	S	O,T	16.7	43.2	40.1	2	690	0	41.7	108.2	45.3
Tolerex	Nestle	FAA	O,T	8	90	2	1	550	0	20	225	2.2
Vital 1.0	Abbott	PB	O,T	16	51	33	1	390	4	40	127	39
Vital 1.5	Abbott	PB	O,T	18	49	33	1.5	610	3.6	45	122.5	39
Vital AF	Abbott	PB	O,T	25	36	39	1.2	425	3.9	62.5	90	43
Vital HN	Abbott	FAA	O,T	16.7	73.8	9.5	1	500	0	41.7	184.5	10.5
Vivonex T.E.N.	Nestle	FAA	T	15	82	3	1	630	0	38	210	2.8
Vivonex Plus	Nestle	FAA	T	18	76	6	1	650	0	45	190	6.7
Vivonex RTF	Nestle	FAA	T	20	70	10	1	630	0	50	175	11.1

*D, diabetic; F, fiber containing; FAA, free amino acid based; HP, high protein; IM, immune modulating; L, liver; P, pulmonary; PB, peptide-based; R, renal; S, standard.

Lactose-free formulas usually use casein and soy as a source of protein; and corn oil, soy oil, and MCT oil as a source of fat. Fiber is not present in most lactose-free formulas, but fiber-enriched products contain between 5 and 15 grams of fiber, as soy polysaccharides, per liter.

"Immune-modulating" formulas supplement their macro- and micronutrient composition with factors (e.g., omega-3 fatty acids, glutamine, antioxidants, arginine) that might affect the response to illness.

Glutamine is used as a fuel by both gut epithelium, hepatocytes and immune cells. Glutamine powder is given at a total dose of 0.3–0.5g/kg/day and should be used with caution in patients with advanced liver disease. Glutamine-enriched formulas appear to improve outcomes in burn and trauma patients.

Omega-3 fatty acids may have anabolic properties in skeletal muscle and affect immune cell activation. Several studies have found that formulas enriched in omega-3 fatty acids reduce mortality and the duration of ventilator requirements in critical illness. In contrast, a recent trial in patients with acute lung injury found that an enteral formula enriched with omega-3 fatty acids worsened outcomes.

Arginine is a key precursor for nitric oxide synthesis and may affect T-cell phenotype and function. Plasma arginine levels decrease early in critical illness however Studies examining the effects of supplemental arginine remain conflicting.

Disease-specific formulas

A number of disease-specific formulas have been designed for patients with specific illnesses.

Hepatic failure

Malnutrition is common in patients with hepatic failure and enteral nutrition is the preferred form of feeding. Protein should not be restricted as a strategy to reduce the risk of hepatic encephalopathy. Branched-chain amino acid formulas have been developed to reduce the risk of hepatic encephalopathy. In critically ill patients, there is little evidence to suggest that these expensive formulas improve outcomes but they may have a role in patients with severe hepatic encephalopathy.

Renal failure

Several specific formulas exist that have reduced amounts of potassium and phosphorous and limited protein content. These formulas may not be appropriate for patients with high protein losses or those receiving continuous dialysis.

Acute pancreatitis

Patients with acute pancreatitis benefit from early (<48 hours) enteral feeding with reductions in infectious morbidity, length of stay and mortality. While gastric feeding can be used, jejunal feeding is preferred in patients who are at high risk for aspiration or who fail to tolerate gastric feeds. There is scant evidence of a benefit of elemental formulas in pancreatitis.

Selection of an appropriate enteral formula

In most patients, a polymeric formula is the cheapest and best tolerated choice. Specific polymeric formulas may be chosen based on the electrolyte and micronutrient needs of the patient. Immune-modulating formulas may be beneficial in patients undergoing major elective surgery, trauma and burn patients but should be used with caution in patients with sepsis. In patients with ARDS and severe acute lung injury, ASPEN recommends use of formulas containing an anti-inflammatory lipid profile.

Implementation of enteral nutrition

All ventilated patients receiving EN should have the head of bed elevated to 30-45 degrees and small bowel feeds should be considered to reduce aspiration risk. Enteral feedings are *contraindicated* in many conditions including persistent nausea or vomiting, intolerable postprandial abdominal pain or diarrhea, mechanical obstruction, ileus, severe malabsorption, use of vasopressors or high output fistulas. Parenteral feeding may be necessary in these cases. Parenteral feeding is also preferred for perioperative nutrition support of malnourished patients.

Parenteral nutrition

PN can be administered through a central vein, central parenteral nutrition (CPN), or a peripheral vein, peripheral parenteral nutrition (PPN). In general CPN is indicated only when a patient has, or is anticipated to be inappropriate to receive sufficient nutrients by the enteral route for more than 7-10 days. Supplementing enteral feeding with parenteral nutrition early (<8 days) in critical illness worsens outcomes and should be avoided (17).

Composition

Protein: Standard solutions are composed of crystalline amino acids in concentrations between 2.75 and 15 per cent. These solutions usually contain 40 to 50 per cent essential and 50 to 60 per cent nonessential amino acids. Most formulas have very little glutamine, glutamate, aspartate, asparaginine, tyrosine, and cysteine.

Carbohydrate: Most formulations use 50–70 per cent dextrose, which is diluted to a final concentration between 15% and 30%. The dextrose in intravenous solutions is hydrated, so each gram of dextrose monohydrate provides 3.4 kcal.

Fat: Lipid emulsions provide fat including the essential fatty acids, linoleic and linolenic acids. These emulsions are usually available as a 20% (2.0 kcal/ml) solution and may be piggy-backed to the other components of TPN. Currently available emulsions contain approximately half to two-thirds of their fatty acids as linoleic acid and approximately 5–10% as linolenic acid. A minimum of ~5% of total calories as a lipid emulsion is necessary to prevent essential fatty acid deficiency. Complications of lipid infusion occur when lipid delivery exceeds 1.0 kcal/kg per hour (0.11 g/kg per hour).

Complications

Many complications have been observed in patients receiving parenteral nutrition.

Hyperglycemia: is common but can be minimized by ensuring that patients are not overfed, using lipid as a calorie source and adding insulin as needed to the TPN. An excellent protocol for glycemic control in patients receiving TPN may be found in a recently published manuscript.

Infectious complications. Catheter-related sepsis is the most common life-threatening complication in patients receiving CPN. Early infections are often caused by S. epidermidis and S. aureus, whereas later infections are often due to gram negative bacteria or fungal species. Meticulous attention to care, glycemic control and avoidance of multilumen catheters reduce infection risk.

Gastrointestinal complications. Hepatic and biliary abnormalities are the most common gastrointestinal complications associated with CPN. Hepatic complications include both biochemical and histological alterations. Biliary complications including acalculous cholecystitis, and cholelithiasis are also common. These complications can be minimized by preventing overfeeding, maintaining glycemic control, preventing line infections, and allowing some enteral feeding if possible.

Clinical management of CPN

Measurement of body weight, fluid intake, and fluid output should be performed daily. Serum electrolytes, phosphorus, and glucose should be measured before and every 1–2 days until stable and then rechecked weekly. If lipid emulsions are being given, serum triglycerides should be evaluated early; concentrations of > 400 mg/dl require reduction of the rate of infusion or discontinuation of lipids. A 0.22 μm filter should be inserted between the intravenous tubing and the catheter when lipid-free CPN is infused and a 1.2 μm filter should be used when a total nutrient admixture containing a lipid emulsion is infused.

Summary

When NS is indicated, EN is generally preferred over CPN. Formula choice is based on metabolic needs, comorbid conditions, and gut structure and function. Patients at risk for aspiration should have the head of the bed elevated and/or receive small bowel feeding. Early use of EN improves outcomes in pancreatitis but is not well established in other conditions. Supplemental glutamine improves outcomes in burn and trauma, the role of other specialized "immunonutrition" formulas remains unclear. When CPN is used, selection of an appropriate mixture of nutrients, meticulous catheter care and avoidance of hyperglycemia can minimize the risk of complications.

Recommended reading

Caesar MP, Mesotten D, Hermans G, Wouters PJ, Schetz M, Meyfroidt G, *et al.* (2011) Early versus late parenteral nutrition in critically ill adults. *The New England Journal of Medicine* Aug.; **365**(6): 506–17.

Dennis MS, Lewis SC, Warlow C (2005) Effect of timing and method of enteral tube feeding for dysphagic stroke patients (FOOD): a multicentre randomised controlled trial. *Lancet* Feb./Mar.; **365**(9461): 764–72.

Gadek JE, DeMichele SJ, Karlstad MD, Pacht ER, Donahoe M, Albertson TE, *et al.* (1999) Effect of enteral feeding with eicosapentaenoic acid, gamma-linolenic acid, and antioxidants in patients with acute respiratory distress syndrome. Enteral Nutrition in ARDS Study Group. *Crit Care Med* Aug.; **27**(8): 1409–20.

Garrel D, Patenaude J, Nedelec B, Samson L, Dorais J, Champoux J, *et al.* (2003) Decreased mortality and infectious morbidity in adult burn patients given enteral glutamine supplements: a prospective, controlled, randomized clinical trial. *Crit Care Med* Oct.; **31**(10): 2444–9.

Ireton-Jones CS, Borman KR, Turner WW, Jr. (1993) Nutrition considerations in the management of ventilator-dependent patients. *Nutr Clin Pract* Apr.; **8**(2): 60–4.

Jakoby MG, Nannapaneni N (2011) An insulin protocol for management of hyperglycemia in patients receiving parenteral nutrition is superior to ad hoc management. *JPEN J Parenter Enteral Nutr* Mar.; **36**(2): 183–8.
Provides practical guidance on glycemic management in patients receiving parenteral nutrition.

Klein S. A primer of nutritional support for gastroenterologists (2002) *Gastroenterology* May; **122**(6): 1677–87.
An excellent and concise overview of nutrition support.

Marchesini G, Bianchi G, Merli M, Amodio P, Panella C, Loguercio C, *et al.* (2003) Nutritional supplementation with branched-chain amino acids in advanced cirrhosis: a double-blind, randomized trial. *Gastroenterology* June; **124**(7): 1792–1801.

McClave SA, Martindale RG, Vanek VW, McCarthy M, Roberts P, Taylor B, *et al.* (2009) Guidelines for the provision and assessment of nutrition support therapy in the adult critically ill patient: Society of Critical Care Medicine (SCCM) and American Society for Parenteral and Enteral Nutrition (A.S.P.E.N.). *JPEN J Parenter Enteral Nutr* May–June; **33**(3): 277–316.
Consensus recommendations for use of nutrition support in many differing medical conditions.

McClave SA, Kushner R, Van Way CW, 3rd, Cave M, DeLegge M, Dibaise J, *et al.* (2011) Nutrition therapy of the severely obese, critically ill patient: summation of conclusions and recommendations. *JPEN J Parenter Enteral Nutr* Sep.; **35**(5 Suppl): 88S–96S.

Pontes-Arruda A, Aragao AM, Albuquerque JD (2006) Effects of enteral feeding with eicosapentaenoic acid, gamma-linolenic acid, and antioxidants in mechanically ventilated patients with severe sepsis and septic shock. *Crit Care Med* Sep; **34**(9): 2325–33.

Rice TW, Wheeler AP, Thompson BT, deBoisblanc BP, Steingrub J, Rock P (2011) Enteral omega-3 fatty acid, gamma-linolenic acid, and antioxidant supplementation in acute lung injury. *Jama* Oct.; **306**(14): 1574–81.

Sato S, Watanabe A, Muto Y, Suzuki K, Kato A, Moriwaki H, *et al.* (2005) Clinical comparison of branched-chain amino acid (l-Leucine, l-Isoleucine, l-Valine) granules and oral nutrition for hepatic insufficiency in patients with decompensated liver cirrhosis (LIV-EN study). *Hepatol Res* Apr; **31**(4): 232–40.

Scheinkestel CD, Kar L, Marshall K, Bailey M, Davies A, Nyulasi I, *et al.* (2003) Prospective randomized trial to assess caloric and protein needs of critically Ill, anuric, ventilated patients requiring continuous renal replacement therapy. *Nutrition* Nov.–Dec; **19**(11–12): 909–16.

Smith GI, Atherton P, Reeds DN, Mohammed BS, Rankin D, Rennie MJ, *et al.* (2010) Dietary omega-3 fatty acid supplementation increases the rate of muscle protein synthesis in older adults: a randomized controlled trial. *The American Journal of Clinical Nutrition* Feb.; **93**(2): 402–12.

Smith GI, Atherton P, Reeds DN, Mohammed BS, Rankin D, Rennie MJ, *et al.* (2011) Omega-3 polyunsaturated fatty acids augment the muscle protein anabolic response to hyperinsulinaemia-hyperaminoacidaemia in healthy young and middle-aged men and women. *Clin Sci (Lond)* Sep.; **121**(6): 267–78.

Wernerman J (2008) Clinical use of glutamine supplementation. *J Nutr* Oct.; **138**(10): 2040S–4S.

Zhou YP, Jiang ZM, Sun YH, Wang XR, Ma EL, Wilmore D (2003) The effect of supplemental enteral glutamine on plasma levels, gut function, and outcome in severe burns: a randomized, double-blind, controlled clinical trial. *JPEN J Parenter Enteral Nutr* July–Aug.; **27**(4): 241–5.

CHAPTER 19

Probiotics

Christina M. Surawicz
Washington University School of Medicine, Seattle, WA, USA

Introduction

Probiotics are living organisms that, when ingested in large enough number, are beneficial to the host. The concept of beneficial organisms dates to over 100 hundred years ago, when the Russian scientist Elie Metchnikoff postulated that lactic acid bacteria could promote longevity, evidently inspired by observing the long life span of Russians in the Caucasus who ate a lot of yogurt. Even before antibiotics had been developed, the German scientist Alfred Nissle isolated a strain of *Escherichia coli* from a World War I soldier who did not develop dysentery while many others around him did. This *E. coli* strain, called *E. coli Nissle* 1917, has been used as a probiotic for many decades. The term "probiotic" became widely used in 1989, when Fuller introduced the idea that they have a beneficial effect on the host. There has been a marked increase in interest in probiotics and their possible health benefit in the western world in the last 20 years due to the appeal of "natural" products (Table 19.1).

The minimum criteria for defining any probiotic is specifying its specific genus and strain, quantifying numbers of viable organisms, confirming they are delivered in adequate numbers to the intestinal tract, with good reliability between batches, and have been found efficacious and safe in human studies.

Probiotics must survive passage through the GI tract, and reach the intestine in viable numbers, and thus should be able to resist gastric acid and bile to reach and colonize the intestine.

Pocket Guide to Gastrointestinal Drugs, Edited by M. Michael Wolfe and Robert C. Lowe. © 2014 John Wiley & Sons, Ltd. Published 2014 by John Wiley & Sons, Ltd.

Table 19.1 Common commercially available probiotic products

Product	Components	CFU count/dose
Culturelle®	*Lactobacillus rhamnosus GG*	10 billion
DanActive® Yogurt	*Lactobacillus casei*	10 billion
Align®	*Bifidobacter infantis*	1 billion
Mutaflor®	*Escherichia coli* Nissle 1917	2–25 billion
VSL #3®	*Bifidobacterium breve, B. longum, B. infantis, Lactobacillus acidophilus, B. plantarum, L. paracasei, L. bulgaricus, Streptococcus thermophilus*	450 billion combined
Yakuit®	*L. casei shirota, B. breve*	6.5 billion
Florastor®	*Saccharomyces boulardii*	5 billion
CFU, colony forming units.		

Pharmacology

Most probiotics are bacteria, commonly Lactobacillus and Bifidobacteria, although one is a yeast (*Saccharomyces boulardii*). Some strains of bacteria have been developed from human sources. Probiotic microbes are characterized by genus and species, and then the specific strain is designated alphanumerically. Some bacterial strains have been genetically engineered to produce immunomodulators, such as interleukin-10.

Lactobacilli are associated with fermented foods such as milk. Many Bifidobacteria are added to foods as probiotic organisms, others are marketed as drugs or food supplements. Because each organism is unique, studies should be conducted with specific strains. For example, results from one strain of Bifidobacteria cannot be generalized to others. Moreover, research should evaluate specific numbers of viable organisms and delivery methods, and efficacy should be confirmed in well-designed randomized controlled trials with adequate numbers of patients enrolled. Unfortunately, many products are marketed without such rigorous research.

Products can contain single organisms or combinations of organisms. Dosing is calculated by colony forming units (CFU), that correlates with the numbers of viable organisms, and which is usually reported as per capsule or by weight of the product. Doses should be based on clinical trials that document efficacy.

Mechanisms of action

The precise mechanisms of action of many probiotics have not been elucidated, and different organisms possess many different properties. However, it is often not known if the mechanisms of action of the organism are actually responsible for the beneficial effect of the probiotics. The properties of organisms include the following:

1 Production of bacteriocins that have antimicrobial action. Lactobacilli are a good example.
2 Production of metabolic products, like short chain fatty acids that are important for colonic health and homeostasis. The probiotic may compete with pathogens for nutrients. Additionally, metabolic products may alter the pH and favor the growth of beneficial organisms.
3 Competitive inhibition of microorganisms (pathogens).
4 Production of enzymes, for example *S. boulardii*, which produces a protease that inactivates the receptor for *C. difficile* Toxin A *in vitro*.
5 Suppression of growth of pathogenic bacteria or preventing epithelial binding and invasion.
6 Improvement of intestinal barrier function by stimulating mucin or by other mechanisms.
7 Modulation of the immune system, such as the production of protective cytokines, which activate local macrophages, increasing secretory IgA among other effects.

Experts suggest that all probiotic bacteria be genetically sequenced. There is a lactic acid bacteria genome sequencing consortium in the USA, and several bifidobacteria strains have been sequenced as well. Genes have been identified that are associated with characteristics that may correlate with efficacy. They correlate with the ability to survive osmotic, acid, bile and oxidative stress. Other genes regulate cell surface factors that may affect adherence, pathogen exclusion, mucosal integrity and host immune factors.

The probiotic manufacturing process is quite variable; functional foods are a rapidly growing market. Most are developed as dairy products, but also as energy bars and dietary supplements. Products can be fermented, freeze dried, lyophilized, and some require refrigeration.

Clinical indications (Table 19.2)

Probiotics have been evaluated in many clinical conditions affecting the GI tracts. There are several excellent reviews (see Ciorba, 2012; Ringel *et al.*, 2012), as well as Cochrane analyses.

Table 19.2 Evidence-based indications for probiotics in GI diseases

	Product	Efficacy
Treatment of infectious diarrhea in children	*Lactobacillus rhamnosus GG* *L. reuteri* ATCC 55730, *L. casei* DN-114001, *S. boulardii*	Moderate
Prevention of infectious diarrhea in children and adults	*Lactobacillus GG,* *L. casei* DN-114001 *S. boulardii*	Weak
Prevention of Traveler's diarrhea	*Lactobacillus GG,* *Saccharomyces boulardii*	Moderate
Prevention of AAD Children and adults	*Lactobacillus GG* *Saccharomyces boulardii*	Strong
Prevention of CDI	Combinations of bacteria	Weak
Treatment of RCDI	*S. boulardii*	Moderate
Pouchitis Prevention Treatment	VSL#3	Strong
IBS	*B. infantis* 35624	Strong
Maintaining remission in Ulcerative colitis	E. coli 1917 Nissle, VSL #3	Moderate
Crohn's	None	None
Prevent NEC	Combinations of bacteria	Moderate

AAD, antibiotic-associated diarrhea; CDI, *Clostridium difficile* infection; IBS, irritable bowel syndrome; NEC, necrotizing enterocolitis; RCDI, recurrent *Clostridium difficile* infection.

Prevention of antibiotic-associated diarrhea (AAD) and *Clostridium difficile* (*C. difficile*) infection

Diarrhea is a frequent side effect of antibiotics and occurs in about 10–20% of patients and is felt to be related to changes in the composition of gut microbiome. Probiotics possess efficacy in the prevention of AAD, especially *Lactobacillus GG* and *S. boulardii,* based on studies in children and in adults. A recent Cochrane analysis of prevention of AAD in adults that evaluated data from sixteen studies looking at a variety of different probiotics, some single strain and some multistrain, reported an overall incidence of AAD of 9% in the probiotic group and 18% in the control group. These results suggest that high-dose probiotics were effective in the prevention of AAD, with a number needed to treat of seven. However, the quality of the evidence was low and imprecise. Similar studies of AAD in adults have also shown a significant decrease in diarrhea with *Saccharomyces boulardii* and *Lactobacillus GG.*

Studies of *C. difficile* infection are much more limited. In smaller trials there were fewer *C. difficile* infections with several probiotics, including *S. boulardii, Clostridium butyricum,* and *Lactobacillus plantarum.* However, the evidence for the effectiveness of these organisms is weak, and at this time they are not recommended for treatment or prevention of *C. difficile* infection (CDI). *S. boulardii* may have a limited role in treating recurrent CDI as an adjunct to antibiotics.

Prevention of infectious diarrhea
Some probiotics have modest efficacy in prevention of infectious diarrhea in children. A meta-analysis of 34 randomized controlled trials evaluating probiotics for the prevention of acute diarrhea did suggest a 35% decrease in infectious diarrhea with multiple probiotics, but their routine use has not been recommended by the American Academy of Pediatrics.

Treatment of infectious diarrhea
Many randomized controlled trials have used various probiotics to treat infectious diarrhea, predominantly in children, with some studies performed in adults. Results have been variable; some lactobacilli decrease symptoms in rotavirus diarrhea, while others do not. Overall, a trend towards a decrease in the duration and severity of diarrhea has been observed, with many probiotics and probiotic mixtures appearing to reduce the duration of infectious diarrhea in children by one day. Studies are limited because of the variety of illnesses, differences in the probiotics used, and diversity in the study methods employed. Overall, the American Academy of Pediatrics concluded that there was evidence to support the use of probiotics early in the course of infectious diarrhea in order to decrease the duration of diarrhea by one day.

Probiotics such as *Lactobacillus GG* have also been used to treat persistent diarrhea. A Cochrane analysis of four relevant trials found that probiotics decreased the severity of diarrhea and also decreased the duration of diarrhea by four days. Nevertheless, the quality of the studies was not sufficient to recommend its use.

Prevention of traveler's diarrhea
A meta-analysis of 12 studies of probiotics for prevention of traveler's diarrhea concluded that both *S. boulardii* and a mixture of *L. acidophilus* and *B. bifidum* appeared to prevent traveler's diarrhea.

Prevention of necrotizing enterocolitis (NEC)
Necrotizing enterocolitis is a severe inflammatory condition that affects low-birth weight infants. It may be infectious in origin and has a high morbidity and mortality. Although there has been considerable interest

in their potential use to prevent NEC, studies in preterm infants have yielded mixed results. Two meta-analyses have concluded that probiotic use is associated with significant benefit in reducing mortality and disease burden. Several probiotics have been tried for prevention, including *Bifidobacterium* species and *Lactobacillus acidophilus*. An updated meta-analysis confirmed their efficacy but cautioned that the optimum probiotic is currently un known and that the long-term effects of these agents requires further study.

Inflammatory bowel disease

Probiotics have been evaluated in the management of inflammatory bowel disease, including both ulcerative colitis and Crohn's disease, which are chronic inflammatory conditions of the intestine. While the use of probiotics, including *E. coli* Nissle strain and VSL #3, in treating ulcerative colitis may provide some benefit, no promising data for the use of probiotics in Crohn's disease have been generated, although several have been evaluated for this condition.

Treatment of pouchitis

Restorative proctocolectomy with ileal pouch-anal anastomosis is the surgical procedure of choice for many patients with ulcerative colitis who require surgery. A common encountered (25–20%) long-term complication is pouchitis, an inflammation of the pouch, which often responds to antibiotic therapy, which is the most common therapy currently employed. Probiotic therapy may represent another viable option. In randomized, controlled trials, VSL-#3 has been shown to both prevent initial episodes of pouchitis postoperatively and to treat pouchitis.

Irritable bowel syndrome

Irritable bowel syndrome is a condition of unknown etiology, although it has been theorized that the condition may occasionally occur as a secondary consequence of intestinal infections. A variety of different treatments, including antispasmotics, diet and probiotics have also been tried. The rationale for probiotics is that the change in gut microbiome might not only change colonic homeostatis, but may also involve immune activation or changes in the neuromuscular function or brain-gut interaction. A probiotic *Bifidobacter infantis* 35624 has been studied in randomized controlled trials and found to improve some of the major symptoms of irritable bowel syndrome, such as abdominal pain, bloating, distension and difficulty in defecation, after 4 weeks of treatment. A systematic review concluded that there was inadequate data on other probiotics (see Brenner *et al.*, 2009).

Helicobacter pylori (*H. pylori*)

Probiotics have also been used as an adjunct to antibiotic therapy in treatment of *H. pylori* infection, with a decrease in side effects. However, their routine use at this time is not recommended.

Constipation

At this time, there is insufficient evidence to recommend probiotics to treat or prevent constipation.

Safety/toxicity

Many of the bacteria normally reside in the human GI tract (*Lactobacillus, Bifidobacteia*), and their safety is thus assumed. However, their safety cannot be assumed, as cases of bacteremia and liver abscess associated with the use of *Lactobacillus GG* have been reported. A review of 72 articles, including randomized controlled trials and case reports, found 20 case reports of adverse events in 32 patients, all being infections with *Lactobacillus* GG or *S. boulardii*. Thus, rigorous safety studies should ideally be performed for all products, but probiotics are currently are not regulated by the FDA, and these studies are thus often not performed. In addition to cases of bacteremia associated with Lactobacilli and fungemia with *S. boulardii*, a recent report of increased mortality from infections and intestinal ischemia in patients with acute severe pancreatitis who had received a probiotic mixture has given clinicians and researchers cause for concern. Another recent report by the Agency for Healthcare Research and Quality (AHRQ) that reviewed 622 studies of probiotics in humans concluded that the relative risk of adverse events was the same as controls. However, it also noted that it is difficult to assess rare adverse events. Given the risks of bacteremia and fungemia, probiotics should probably not be used in immune suppressed individuals.

Because these agents are not regulated by the FDA, they have not been classified in pregnancy or in children, but there are no guidelines that guide the use of probiotics in either pregnancy or in children.

Summary

Probiotics are appealing options for the treatment of gastrointestinal diseases; they are naturally occurring, and different strains possess different mechanisms of action that may explain their efficacy. The two best well-studied indications are probiotics to prevent antibiotic-associated diarrhea in children and adults and to treat infectious diarrhea in children. Additionally, studies of probiotics to prevent infectious diarrhea in children and traveler's diarrhea in adults suggest possible benefit, and the role of probiotics to prevent necrotizing enterocolitis is also promising, although further trials are needed. There is preliminary evidence that probiotics may be beneficial in the treatment of ulcerative colitis and in the prevention and treatment of pouchitis, but no evidence for a role in Crohn's disease has been determined to date. Interest in probiotics to treat irritable bowel syndrome is great, and some products may provide benefit in treating bloating and pain. While probiotics are generally safe, they should not be used in immunosuppressed individuals due to the risks of bacteremia and fungemia.

Recommended reading

AlFaleh K, Anabrees J, Bassler D, Al-Kharfi T (2011) Probiotics for prevention of necrotizing enterocolitis in preterm infants. *Cochrane Database Syst Rev* CD005496.

Allen SJ, Masrtinez EG, Gregorio GV, Dans LF (2010) Probiotics for treating acute infectious diarrhoea. *Cochrane Database Syst Rev* **10**: CD003048.

Bernaola Aponte G, Bada Macilla CA, Pariasca C, *et al.* (2010) Probiotics for treating persistent diarrhoea in children. *Cochrane Database Syst Rev* **11**: CD007401.

Besselink MG, van Santvoort HC, Buskens E, *et al.* (2008) Probiotic prophylaxis in predicted severe acute pancreatitis: a randomized, double-blind, placebo-controlled trial. *Lancet* **371**: 851.

Brenner DM, Moeller MJ, Chey WD, Schoenfeld PS (2009) The utility of probiotics in the treatment of irritable bowel syndrome: a systematic review. *Am J Gastroenterol* **104**: 1033–49.

Butterworth AD, Thomas AG, Akobeng AK (2008) Probiotics for treatment of active Crohn's disease. *Cochrane Summaries* CD006634.

Chmielewska A, Szajewska H (2010) Systematic review of randomized controlled trials: probiotics for functional constipation. *World J Gastorenterol* **16**: 69.

Ciorba MA (2012) Perspectives in clinical gastroenterology and hepatology. A Gastroenterologist's guide to probiotics. *Clin Gastroenterol Hepatol* **10**: 960–8.

Deshpande G, Rao S, Patole S, Bulsara M (2010) Updated meta-analysis of probiotics for preventing necrotizing enterocolitis in preterm neonates. *Pediatrics* **125**: 921–30.

Gordon NK, Fagbemi AO, Thomas AG, Akobeng AK (2011) Probiotics for maintenance of remission in ulcerative colitis. *Cochrane Summaries* CD007443.

Guandalini S (2011) Probiotics for prevention and treatment of diarrhea. *J Clin Gastroenterol* **45**: S149–51.

Guarner F, Khan AG, Garisch J, *et al.* (2011) Probiotics and prebiotics. *World Gastroenterology Organization Global Guidelines*. www.worldgastroenterology.org/…/Probiotics_FINAL_20111128.pd.
This excellent review prepared for the World Gastroenterology Organization outlines the role of prebiotics and probiotics and provides an excellent overview.

Hempel S, Newberry S, Ruelaz A, *et al.* (2011) Safety of probiotics used to reduce risk and prevent or treat disease. Evidence Report/Technology Assessment No. 200. *This paper is an expert review looking at safety of probiotics for prevention and treatment of various diseases and is an important review of an area that requires more study.*

Hempel S, Newberry SJ, Maher AR, Wang Z, Miles JN, Shanman, *et al.* (2012) Probiotics for the prevention and treatment of antibiotic-associated diarrhea: a systematic review and meta-analysis. *JAMA* **307**: 1959–69.

Holubar SD, Cima RR, Sandborn WJ, Pardi DA (2012) Treatment and prevention of pouchitis after ileal pouch-anal anastomosis for chronic ulcerative colitis. *Cochrane Database Syst Rev* CD001176.

Johnston BC, Goldenberg JZ, Vandvik PO, Sun X, Guyatt GH (2011) Probiotics for the prevention of pediatric antibiotic-associated diarrhea. *Cochrane Database Syst Rev* CD004827.

Lesbros-Pantoflickova D, Corthésy-Theulaz I, Blum AL (2007) Helicobacter pylori and probiotics. *J Nutr* **137**: 812S–818S.

Mallon P, McKay D, Kirk S, Gardiner K (2007) Probiotics for induction of remission in ulcerative colitis. *Cochrane Database Syst Rev* CD005573.

McFarland LV (2006) Meta-analysis of probiotics for the prevention of antibiotic associated diarrhea and the treatment of *Clostridium difficile* disease. *Am J Gastroetnerol* **101**: 812.

McFarland LV (2007) Meta-analysis of probiotics for the prevention of traveler's diarrhea. *Travel Med Infect Dis* **5**: 97. *This manuscript represents the only meta-analysis available analyzing the role of probiotics for prevention of traveler's diarrhea.*

Nelson RL, Kelsey P, Leeman, Neardon N, Patel H, Paul K, *et al.* (2011) Antibiotic treatment for *Clostridium difficile*-associated diarrhea in adults. *Cochrane Summaries* DOI:10.1002/14651858.CD004610.

Quigley EMM (2007) Probiotics in irritable bowel syndrome: an immunomodulatory strategy? *J Am College of Nutrition* **26**: 584S–690S.

Ringel Y, Quigley EMM, Lin HC (2012) Using probiotics in gastrointestinal disorders. *Am J Gastroenterol Suppl* **1**: 34–40.

Ritchie ML, Romanuk TN (2012) A meta-analysis of probiotic efficacy for gastrointestinal diseases. *PLosONE* **7** (334938). doi:10.1371/journal.pone/0034938. *This is an excellent overview meta-analysis of the role of various probiotics for various gastrointestinal diseases. It is quite comprehensive and very up-to-date.*

Sazawal S, Hiermath G, Dhingra U, *et al.* Efficacy of probiotics in prevention of acute diarrhoea: a meta-analysis of masked, randomized, placebo-controlled trials. *Lancet Infect Dis* **6**: 374.

Segarra-Newnham M. Probiotics for *Clostridium difficile*-associated diarrhea: focus on *Lactobacillus rhamnosus GG* and *Saccharomyces boulardii*. *Annals of Pharmacotherapy* **41**: 1212–21.

Shen B (2012) Acute and chronic pouchitis – pathogenesis, diagnosis and treatment. *Nat Rev Gastroenterol Hepatol* **9**: 323–33.

Thomas DW, Greer FR (2010) Committee on Nutrition. Clinical Report – Probiotics and prebiotics in pediatrics. *Pediatrics* **125**: 1217–27.

Videlock EJ, Cremonini F (2012) Meta-analysis: probiotics in antibiotic-associated diarrhoea. *Aliment Pharmacol Ther* **35**: 1355.

Wang Q, Dong J, Zhu Y (2012) Probiotic supplement reduces risk of necrotizing enterocolitis and mortality in preterm very low-birth-weight infants: an updated meta-analysis of 20 randomized, controlled trials. *J Pediatr Srug* **47**: 241–8.

Whelan K, Myers CE (2010) Safety of probiotics inpatient receiving nutritional support: a systematic review of case reports, randomized controlled trials, and nonrandomized trials. *Am J Clin Nutr* **91**: 687–703.

Whorwell PJ, Altringer L, Morel J, Bond Y, Charbonneau D, O'Mahony L, *et al.* (2006) Efficacy of an encapsulated probiotic *Bifidobacterium infantis* 35624 in women with irritable bowel syndrome. *Am J Gastroenterol* **101**: 1581–90.

Index

Pocket Guide to Gastrointestinal Drugs, Edited by M. Michael Wolfe and Robert C. Lowe. © 2014
John Wiley & Sons, Ltd. Published 2014 by John Wiley & Sons, Ltd.